Sensual Religion

Religion and the Senses
Series Editor: Graham Harvey, The Open University, UK

Everyday and/or vernacular religions are now at the cutting edge of the study of religions. The agenda of Religious Studies as well as that of other disciplines which overlap in some aspects with the study of religion (e.g. Classics, History, Sociology, Anthropology and [in some places] Philosophy) has been revitalised by this focus on lived reality. This resonates with the growing interest in materiality and embodiment which have both provoked 'turns' in academic debate and teaching. Criticisms, however, have been levelled against the ways in which 'materiality' does not always engage with materials (stuff) and 'embodiment' sometimes suggests the priority of some interiority (mind, agency, etc.).

The proposed series aims to push further the project of placing lived, material and bodily religion at the definitive centre of studies of religion(s). It will do this by foregrounding bodily sensation and material practice as religion (rather than expressions, experiences or representations of something prior to bodies, acts and things). It develops the interdisciplinary conversation encouraged by Paul Stoller's *Sensuous Scholarship* (1997) and, especially, presents and promotes research about real life religion approached through performative and materialist methods, as illustrated by, e.g., Manuel Vasquez's *More than Belief* (2011) and Graham Harvey's *Food, Sex and Strangers* (2013).

Forthcoming:

Religion and Sight
Edited by Louise Child and Aaron Rosen

Sensual Religion

Religion and the Five Senses

Edited by
Graham Harvey and Jessica Hughes

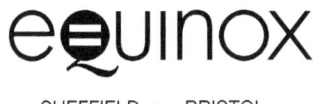

SHEFFIELD UK   BRISTOL CT

Published by Equinox Publishing Ltd.
UK: Office 415, The Workstation, 15 Paternoster Row, Sheffield, South Yorkshire S1 2BX
USA: ISD, 70 Enterprise Drive, Bristol, CT 06010

www.equinoxpub.com

Chapters 1, 3, 5, 7 and 9 first published in Volume 2.1 of the journal *Body and Religion*.
Chapters 2, 4, 6, 8 and 10 first published in Volume 2.2 of the journal *Body and Religion*.
© Equinox Publishing Ltd 2018

First published in book form 2018
© Graham Harvey, Jessica Hughes and contributors 2018

All rights reserved. No part of this publication may be reproduced or transmitted in any form or by any means, electronic or mechanical, including photocopying, recording or any information storage or retrieval system, without prior permission in writing from the publishers.

British Library Cataloguing-in-Publication Data
A catalogue record for this book is available from the British Library.

ISBN-13   978 1 78179 414 2   (hardback)
          978 1 78179 415 9   (paperback)
          978 1 78179 681 8   (ePDF)

Library of Congress Cataloging-in-Publication Data
Names: Harvey, Graham, 1959 – editor.
Title: Sensual religion : religion and the five senses / edited by Graham Harvey and Jessica Hughes.
Description: Bristol : Equinox Publishing Ltd., 2018. | Series: Religion and the senses | Includes bibliographical references and index.
Identifiers: LCCN 2017058417 (print) | LCCN 2018025869 (ebook) | ISBN 9781781796818 (ePDF) | ISBN 9781781794142 (hb) | ISBN 9781781794159 (pb)
Subjects: LCSH: Senses and sensation—Religious aspects. | Human body—Religious aspects.
Classification: LCC BL65.B63 (ebook) | LCC BL65.B63 S47 2018 (print) | DDC 203—dc23
LC record available at https://lccn.loc.gov/2017058417

Typeset by S.J.I. Services, New Delhi
Printed and bound by Lightning Source Inc. (La Vergne, TN), Lightning Source UK Ltd. (Milton Keynes), Lightning Source AU Pty. (Scoresby, Victoria).

Contents

Series Foreword   vii
Graham Harvey

List of Figures   x

Introduction   1
Graham Harvey

Section One: Smell

1 A Pleasing Odour for Yahweh: The Smell of Sacrifices on Mount Gerizim and in the Hebrew Bible   19
Anne Katrine de Hemmer Gudme

2 Wafting Incense and Heavenly Foods: The Importance of Smell in Chinese Religion   37
Shawn Arthur

Section Two: Taste

3 The Taste of Religion in the Roman World   63
Zena Kamash

4 Candomblé's Eating Myths: Religion Stated in Food Language   84
Patricia Rodrigues de Souza

Section Three: Sight

5   Sight and the Byzantine Icon   109
    Angeliki Lymberopoulou

6   'Seeing' My Beloved: *Darśan* and the Sikhi Perspective   131
    Opinderjit Kaur Takhar

Section Four: Hearing

7   Resounding Mysteries: Sound and Silence in the Eleusinian Soundscape   149
    Georgia Petridou

8   North American Indigenous Song, the Sacred and the Senses   170
    Byron Dueck

Section Five: Touch

9   The Texture of the Gift: Religious Touching in the Greco-Roman World   191
    Jessica Hughes

10   Touching, Crafting, Knowing: Religious Artefacts and the Fetish within Animism   215
    Amy Whitehead

Index   237

Series Foreword

GRAHAM HARVEY

Religion is sensual because it is corporeal and earthy. Religion is something that people (always bodies) do in the world (always physical). It is seen, heard, tasted, smelled and touched, and often involves senses of place, decency, awe, humour, value and honour. These and other senses work together (although not always successfully), and they are integral to corporeality and to engagement with the world. Some of our experiences privilege particular senses – as when we close our eyes to better appreciate music. The sensual impact of religious activities can be staged to employ or heighten one sense at a time, perhaps allowing incense or singing to take a lead. Or they can work together as when the burning of incense coincides with the ringing of bells to direct attention. There are myriad ramifications. This series engages with a wide range of such matters.

It is true that some religions make the physical senses a battleground: encouraging the suppression of bodily senses and desires in favour of 'more spiritual' leanings. In doing so, they do not contradict the assertion that religion is sensual but, rather, they evidence it. Progress in seeking putatively non-material gains or experiences, or in seeking mystical and transcendent states, may be recognised by degrees of success in restraining the more everyday senses. If these senses are not restrained, they may be trained to serve 'more elevated' purposes. Paying attention to the feeling of inward and outward breathing to initiate mindfulness does not negate sensuality but employs it. The banning of music creates alternative sonic environments (e.g. of silence or spoken words) that are deemed suitable to the feel of some ways of being religious. Similarly, quasi-cyborg interactions in online and virtual religion do not challenge the sensuality of religious activities but are conducted through the touch of keyboards, sight of screens and hearing of digital sounds. Examples could be multiplied.

This series has deep foundations in approaches to religion which emphasise the everyday, practice or performance, materiality, embodiment and affect. It owes much to the scholarship of religion and gender which brings into sharp focus the importance of attending to lived realities and refuses to waft away the stench of patriarchal power dynamics. *Religion and the Senses* begins with the assumption that religion is something people do. For some people, this 'doing of religion' is especially about cognition: the encouragement of correct believing or correct understanding. These activities have been emphasised by scholars as well as religious practitioners in most publications about religion. However, religion is as much about the preparation, eating and waste-management of the foods people eat or avoid as it is about the putative meanings of food-rules. Communities are made by eating together, sharing appropriate foods at appropriate times, and equally by avoiding inappropriate foods and those who eat them. They may be riven by the wearing of the wrong costume or by visual or auditory attention to inappropriate media. Religious conflicts can be less about differences of belief than about the censorial setting apart of sensory worlds.

Religion and the Senses builds on these relatively familiar perspectives on lived religion. However, the series is more than summative of existing knowledge. It seeks to advance the cutting edge of debates. It is provocative because it engages with the sensuality of religion on the understanding that religion is *fully* sensual, corporeal and earthy. It pushes further an existing project in which religious senses largely serve to enhance appreciation of the lived reality of religions. Great advances in understanding and analysing religion have been made. However, just as debates about 'materiality' have not always engaged with materials (stuff) and those about 'embodiment' have sometimes suggested the priority of some interiority (mind, agency, etc.), so those about religion and the senses have sometimes suggested that 'religion' exists before and apart from senses. In the books which comprise *Religion and the Senses*, religion will be pursued as something that is not merely represented by or expressed in sensual data (e.g. arts and acts), but is a matter of bodies moving through the world. Attending to sensuality does not (merely) add colour and drama to our views of religion(s). It is not only about the vignettes that introduce our debates. Religion is the smelling, tasting, touching, hearing and seeing of the world in particular ways. We need to attend to everything from bodily affects to trained enculturation (not to evoke a nature/culture dualism but to indicate a rich diversity of topics) in order to understand how sensual religion propels people in their daily and ritual negotiations with life.

This foreword has made use of the conventional idea that there are five senses, albeit with some recognition that these can or must work together (sometimes conflictually). However, the series is not restricted to discussion of those five senses or their synaesthetic interactions. These are our entry points, our 'starting from where we are' places. The journey towards a richer and fuller sense of religion will entail a much wider notion of senses. It will require us to explore senses of place, decorum, decency, value, health/well-being, the uncanny, humour, honour and others. These 'extra' senses provide even greater possibilities for considering movement, relationships, interactions, locations and other matters.

Some of these 'senses' might make more immediate sense than others – e.g. sense of place is a relatively familiar theme in discussing religious locations and commitments. Sense of value encourages consideration of religion and economic systems (e.g. capitalist, gift, votive and sacrificial economies), charity or philanthropy, and of ultimate versus putatively lesser 'needs' or concerns. Sense of decorum might bring discussions of religion and costume into dialogue with discussions of religious discipline and deportment (e.g. stipulations that elders should not run, children should be silent, women should be humble). Sense of honour can generate acts of violence against perceived wrong-doers as well as celebration of specific practices. The sense of the uncanny brings us face-to-face with the worlds of possession and ghosts, with feelings of unease or dread that may require the employment of religious specialists. In contrast with sense of place perhaps the sense of the uncanny is about dislocation and unease in the presence of the unknown, unexpected or unwelcome. As these presences are sometimes faced with edgy trickster tales, they provide an additional reason (if we needed it) to immerse ourselves in the sense of humour. If nothing else, jokes told within a religion (about that religion or about others) are revelatory of what is truly at the heart of that lifeway. Reiterating the synaesthetic and corporeal nature of all the senses, perhaps these religious jokes sometimes provoke throaty chortles or 'belly laughs'. Engaging with these many and varied, but usually interacting, senses will require authors and readers to confront a broad spectrum of religious acts and ideas, some more edgy or contested than others.

There are, in short, many good reasons for studying religion and the senses, including the assertion made by this foreword (and contested both by some religionists and perhaps within some of the following chapters) that religion is fully and definitively sensual, corporeal and worldly. This series takes up the project of the 'turns' to lived religion, everyday religion, materiality, gender, embodiment and performance. By sustained focus on the senses – perhaps mediating mechanisms between our bodies and our world – we will gain a greatly improved sense of what religion is and what religious people do.

List of Figures

1.1 and 1.2 Passover sacrifice on Mount Gerizim	22
2.1 The typical Chinese practice of 'lighting incense and prostrating'	39
2.2 Cloud of incense on Mt Qingcheng, Sichuan, China	45
2.3 Types of incense, Xi'an, China	48
2.4 A selection of Chinese incense boxes	55
3.1 Tripole graph showing percentages of domestic ox, sheep/goat and pig for all site types in Roman Britain	69
3.2 Tripole graph showing percentages of domestic ox, sheep/goat and pig for Romano-British temple sites	70
3.3 The final phase of the Crypta Balbi *mithraeum* animal assemblage by percentage of fragment count	78
3.4 The animal bone assemblage from the seventh century CE occupation at Crypta Balbi by percentage of fragment count	79
4.1 *Ifá* divination board with cowry shells	87
4.2 *Opele*, made with palm tree seeds	88
4.3 *Borí* ritual: initiate surrounded by votive foods	91
4.4 Candomblé priestess giving a devotee a popcorn bath	97
5.1 Panel painting of the Virgin *Hodegetria*, fifteenth century (?)	110
5.2 Wall painting of *The Mandylion*, 1319, Crete	115
5.3 Wall painting depicting hell scenes, 1372, Crete	119

List of Figures

5.4	Interior view of the church of Hosios Loukas, eleventh century, Greece	120
5.5	The Entry into Jerusalem, eleventh century (?), ivory	122
5.6	Nativity, fourteenth-century wall painting, Crete	125
6.1	*Kirtan* in a gurdwara in the UK	133
6.2	Pizza *langar* at Guru Nanak Gurdwara, Wolverhampton	134
7.1	Drawing of a hydria (the 'Regina Vasorum') from Cumae, now in the Hermitage Museum, St. Petersburg	155
7.2	Drawing of the Ninnion Tablet, c. 370 BCE	156
7.3	Map of the Eleusinian sanctuary	160
8.1	Fancy Shawl dancers performing at Manito Ahbee 2016 International Pow Wow	173
8.2	Drum group performing at Manito Ahbee 2016 International Pow Wow	174
9.1	Red-figured South Italian hydria showing the assault of the priestess Cassandra by the Lesser Ajax in the temple of Athena at Troy, 340–320 BCE	192
9.2	Marble votive relief showing Asklepios healing via touch. c. 350 BCE, from the Asklepieion at Piraeus	199
9.3	Marble stele of Meidon, first–second century CE	201
9.4	White marble stele of Diokles, from the sanctuary of Zeus Sabazios and Meter Hipta in Kula	204
9.5	Calyx krater depicting Apollo and his sister Artemis killing the children of Niobe, Orvieto, 460–450 BCE	206
9.6	Stele depicting Apollo Bozenos with his axe, from Kula	207
9.7	Confession stele showing the god Men holding a sceptre, from the territory of Saittai in Lydia, 164–165 CE	209
10.1	The Virgin of Alcala	217
10.2	'Going under the mantle' of the Virgin of Alcala	220
10.3	Under the white mantle	228

Introduction

GRAHAM HARVEY

Religions are the causes and contexts of an extravagant diversity of sensual forms and experiences. This book initiates a series in which relationships between senses and religion are given the attention they deserve. By presenting studies of particular religious practices and communities the contributors invite us to reflect on the ways in which religion involves sensuality (diverse bodily practices, experiences and engagements). Similarly, by focusing on particular senses, and relationships between different senses, the authors also encourage us to improve our understanding of the ways in which religions are lived and performed. This will lead us to notice things we had previously missed, or to think about seemingly familiar material in new and fresh ways. This book, and the series it initiates, entail and expand a vibrantly interdisciplinary and trans-disciplinary project. They bring different approaches, methods and perspectives to bear on exciting debates. Their primary ambition is to push for a more radical and sustained engagement with the bodily, performative and material living of religion than has yet happened.

The purpose of this introduction is to set out the key features of this book. It begins with an orientation to terms such as 'senses', 'sensual' and 'sensorium'. Then it evokes examples of the sensual dynamics of religions, making use of selected cosmological, creation or origins narratives to highlight some of the many possibilities for conceiving of sensory relations with the world. Finally, it provides an overview of the ways in which the chapters engage with the five senses of smell, taste, sight, hearing and touch. It will set out our reasons for selecting these senses and our reasons for selecting particular religious examples or case studies.

SENSES, THE SENSORIUM AND THE SENSORIAL WORLD

The term 'senses' identifies mechanisms through which bodies gain and integrate knowledge about the world around them. Senses of smell, taste, sight, hearing and touch are just some of the ways in which we know the world. The contexts of our movements through life are made known to us by the interrelated working of these and other senses (some of which will be introduced below). The combination of senses can be called the 'sensorium'. It is vital to appreciate that there is a continuous negotiation between the senses, none of them working alone, but some dominating over others for a period, and some working more harmoniously with others in particular circumstances. Sometimes the 'working together' is so close that we are not aware of which predominates. This is particularly true of our senses of smell and taste, but some people see sounds and experience other forms of synaesthesia (a term for various fusions of senses). Also, when one sense (e.g. sight) is impaired, another (e.g. hearing) might compensate to gain and processes knowledge of what is happening. The senses and the full sensorium can be manipulated so that on occasions, or throughout life, people can be more or less attentive to particular sensations. Indeed, one of the causes of cultural diversity is the privileging of one or more senses over others. Sight, for instance, is often treated as more trustworthy and/or informative than other senses (e.g. in the phrase 'seeing is believing'). Religious communities often involve training in diminishing attention to distractions coming from most senses in order to concentrate on the words people are meant to hear, the sights we are meant to observe, or the feeling of our breathing as we meditate. Much of what we will encounter in this and future volumes of this series arises from the ever-shifting interplay between the 'working together' and the privileging of different senses.

We are not only beings who *have* senses or the equipment to sense the world. We are not inhabitants of physical bodies. We are sensate or sensual beings. We are hubs of relationships between senses and worldly, physical, sensual phenomena. Describing both bodies and the world as 'sensual' reminds us that the world is not 'out there' beyond our bodies but it penetrates and infuses our bodies as smells, tastes, sights, sounds and feelings reach our noses, tongues, eyes, ears and skin – and the receptors and nerves which absorb them. Our bodies, our 'we', our relational selves, are in their element, continuously moving through and being moved through that which can be sensed by these five and other senses. The world is sensual or sensorial, full of smells, tastes, sights, sounds and textures. Having evolved on this planet, we fit well with it. Our senses meet that which can be sensed. We can smell what can be smelled, taste what can be tasted, see what can be seen, hear what can be heard, and feel what can be felt. Our sensate carnality is part of the sensorial materiality of the world, and both are in continuous sensual relationship. Once again, however, note that our cultural contexts and other factors can significantly affect whether we do actually become aware of the myriad possibilities through which we move. There is continuous reciprocity between the sensorium that is bodied as humans, the sensorial world in which we participate, and the ways in which we have been shaped by upbringing, life-choices, previous experience and other relational pressures or encouragements. (David Abram's *The Spell of the Sensuous*, 1996, evokes and discusses much of this in inspiring detail.)

In fact, we are continuously sensing far more than we are consciously aware of or attentive to. However, we can deliberately employ additional filtering mechanisms when we concentrate to try to smell one rose in a garden, to taste one spice in a curry, to see some detail of a painting, to hear a particular bird-song, or to feel the texture of a fabric. Sometimes pungent smells, strong tastes, bright lights, loud noises or sharp pain can overwhelm us. Many of us have also had the experience of realising that we have not noticed a sound, smell, taste, sight or feeling that has been there all along. Once we do notice such things, our senses can be focused on them. We can be transformed or the world can be transformed for us. Religions and other aspects of culture (e.g. art, politics, science, sport, catering) all utilize the relations between sensorium and sensuality. They emphasise one or more senses over others. They deny the value of some senses on some occasions, presenting them as distractions from what, they claim, should be more important focuses. Religions, in particular, seem to encourage either excesses or frugality of sensuality. Evidence for this may be gleaned from the fact that one synonym of 'sensual', namely 'voluptuous', is rarely if ever used in religious contexts. Examples of these and other sensory engagements and exclusions in religions will be explored further in the chapters and books which follow.

SENSUAL COSMOLOGIES AND ORATORY

The cosmological, origins and creation narratives of religions perform many roles. They may, for example, have didactic functions in shaping understandings of the world or in moulding ways of behaving. They may entertain as well as construct communities as they are told and responded to. Whatever their role, their impact is certainly heightened by the sensuality woven through the stories. Many of them also indicate, sometimes in surprising ways, that a lack of sensuality or a diminished sensorium is problematic. The following consideration of such matters provides one way of evoking relationships between religion and the senses.

Reading the opening words of great religious epics, even in translation, can be deeply affective. Here is how the Akkadian *Enuma Elish* (a three thousand year old text from what is now Iraq) begins:[1] 'When in the heights, the sky above was not named, and earth beneath did not yet bear a name ...'. Not even the basic sounds with which things and relations are named had been heard. There were only waters, the sweet-tasting waters named Apsû, and the salt waters named Tiamat. In their chaotic mingling they gave birth to a host of deities whose loud clamour became irritating and provoked a series of violent conflicts within the primordial dysfunctional family. Eventually, the body parts of the first parents were used to construct the cosmos, the homes of deities, and the work places of humans. The narrative is replete with sensuality, referring, for example, to the smell of incense and ruptured entrails, the taste of the waters and of beer, the brightness of the moon and of faces beaming with joy, and the tactile surveying of the world and of strong walls. It is, however, hearing that predominates. Beginning with the absence of names, the *Enuma Elish* tells us of the clamour of deities, of Tiamat's silence and then rage when confronted with Apsû's plot, of various counsels of war, of decrees and commands, of the incantation of spells, of declarations of praise, of the naming of weapons and houses, and finally of the reverent calling out of the fifty names of the god Marduk.

The *Epic of Gilgamesh* (a four thousand year old text from Uruk, also in what is now Iraq) tells us that sound was also a problem in a later phrase of this cosmic story.[2] Having expected to be able to relax once they had made humans to do all the work, the deities who had annoyed their parents by being noisy now became irritated by the clamour of their increasingly numerous servants. After a flood intended to wash away the trouble subsided, a survivor, Utnapishtim, offered libations and sacrifices to the deities who, smelling the 'sweet savour', gathered around 'like flies'. Similarly, the deity in *Breshīt/Genesis*, the Jewish and Christian account of the first

---

1   The following evocation paraphrases the translations made by Leonard King (1902) and Wilfred Lambert (2007).
2   See George (2003) for an accessible expert translation.

shaping of the world, smelled the sacrifice offered by Noah after he survived a flood. This narrative, too, begins with a confused and chaotic initial state: 'without form and void', with 'darkness over the face of the deep'. All is changed when the creative deity speaks. Although the rest of the narrative emphasises sight (e.g. in the refrain that the deity 'saw that it was good' at each stage of his work), it is the speaking/hearing of the words 'Let there be light' which propels the narrative and creation onwards towards an incremental increase of order in the cosmos. The narrative resonates strongly with later biblical passages that insist (perhaps compulsively) on orderly separations between different kinds of cattle, crops, cloth, people, places and practices. Everything in its place and a place for everything seems to be the rule.

This sense of orderliness is tested in the 'Garden of Eden' section of the *Breshīt/Genesis* narrative. Here we encounter humans discovering a sense of shame at being naked and a sense of loss on being removed from the cosy kindergarten of their orchard paradise. Perhaps the authors also expect us to respond with a sense of humour to the idea of a snake who can not only talk temptingly but is also reduced to crawling on its belly (as if crawling was not just what serpents do). Before the first humans and that first snake leave the primordial garden, the text seems to encourage us to imagine them and their creator in a rich sensual domain of shade and light, blossom and fruit, breezes and bird-song, and the touch of tree-bark and nourishing soil.

An initial absence of noise, the establishment of a sensually pleasing order, irritation with noise, and then the divine smelling of offerings unite these diverse tales. Perhaps this points to shared cultural understandings of the senses across the West Asian region. To be clear, these narratives do not begin with an absence of things (or with a nothingness) but with a chaotic mingling of stuff. It is sound which interrupts this state and initiates the processes of re-structuring which allows for an explosion of the visual, tactile, olfactory, gustatory and other senses with which deities, humans and all beings engage with the world. That the deities and humans utilise their senses differently (humans tasting food, deities smelling it) is also an important indicator that we should not think of the relationship between religion and the senses as a simple matter.

The opening lines of Hesiod's *Theogony* (a Greek epic from nearly three thousand years ago) also privilege hearing but link sound to movement, fusing senses of touch and balance:

> From the Heliconian Muses let us begin to sing, who hold the great and holy mount of Helicon, and dance on soft feet about the deep-blue spring and the altar of the almighty son of Cronos, and, when they have washed their tender bodies in Permessus or in the Horse's Spring or Olmeius, make their fair, lovely dances upon highest Helicon and move with vigorous feet. Thence they arise and go abroad by night, veiled in thick mist, and utter their song with lovely voice, praising [...] the holy race of all the [...] deathless ones that are for ever. And one day they taught Hesiod glorious song while he was shepherding his lambs under holy Helicon .... (Evelyn-White 1914)

Hesiod is spoken to by these dancing 'ready-voiced daughters of great Zeus', given a rod 'of sturdy laurel' and has a 'divine voice' breathed into him so that he can sing of the deities and the muses. Perhaps we need to re-read the previous narratives to determine whether the hearing of sounds should also sometimes, often or always suggest a sense of touch as the Muses' 'soft feet' dance on mountains and their 'tender bodies' are washed in springs. In *Breshīt/Genesis* the deity who is heard 'hovers' over the deep chaotic waters. The clamour of deities and humans is not produced by static bodies but by those in contact with the materials of the cosmos and the earth. Voices and labour combine to generate senses of irritation in others. There is probably more to notice about the interaction of senses. Hesiod, for example, also points to the suppression of the sense of sight as the Muses 'go abroad by night, veiled in thick mist', heard but not seen. In many religious traditions, divine and other-worldly beings are hidden from sight unless they choose to reveal themselves. They seem more at ease with being heard than with any other sense – but perhaps that idea needs to be tested as this series of books seeks deeper understanding of the relationships between religions and senses.

Certainly, however, deprivation of the senses is also a theme in the Mayan *Popol Vuh* (a Quiché-Maya codex from the mid-sixteenth century, based on earlier texts). After a long preamble, the writers tell us about the state of things before creation began. This sets the scene for telling us why the deities wanted to make the world and its inhabitants.

> This is the account of when all is still silent and placid. All is silent and calm. Hushed and empty is the womb of the sky. These, then, are the first words, the first speech. There is not yet one person, one animal, bird, fish, crab, tree, rock, hollow, canyon, meadow, or forest. All alone the sky exists. The face of the earth has not yet appeared. Alone lies the expanse of the sea, along with the womb of all the sky. There is not yet anything gathered together. All is at rest. Nothing stirs. All is languid, at rest in the sky. There is not yet anything standing erect. Only the expanse of the water, only the tranquil sea lies

alone. There is not yet anything that might exist. All lies placid and silent in the darkness, in the night. (Christenson 2007: 58)

Imagine the choices made by the authors: crabs, canyons, meadows .... Perhaps they crafted their narratives while smelling the sea, or while feeling breezes climbing and descending mountain slopes, or while hearing the wind in the corn. But they imagine a time when there was only light. There is sight but no object to catch the eye, only an expanse and a flatness. There is no movement. There is no noise, no words. There is only stasis and silence. The authors go on to evoke the great yearning of the world's makers which inspires them to make beings (eventually humans) who can praise and venerate them. The noise of praise songs and speeches is a cause for creation. Processions and prostrations of bodies are causes for world-making. The ability to communicate with and learn from experience and from others are causes of world-making. These (noises and movements) are what supports the lives of deities. Fully sensual bodies and a rich sensorial cosmos are necessary to the relationship between deities, humans and everything else which exists.

Imagine that all these tales, and all the others, were not only shaped for sonorous telling but have evolved as orators declaim, proclaim and exclaim them. What locations do these orators perform in? In acoustically rich halls with careful lighting? By fires at night, with cool breezes at their backs and flickering light in their eyes? How do they move their hands to emphasise a word, a point, a movement in the tale or its telling? Do they make eye-contact with their audiences while reciting? Do they signal improvisations by a change of tone or a sudden shifting of their posture? Do they offer libations before they pick up the traces of ancestral tales? Are their words and gestures accompanied by perfumed incense or background music? Do their audiences join in at well known moments or refrains? Do they gasp with astonishment or applaud with pleasure? Even in their written forms, these narratives involve not only choices of words but also of tone and pace – along with an ear for drama and a sense of occasion. They remain sensually rich and derive continuing power from this.

As a final example, for now, of an origins narrative replete with sensory references, imagine listening to a contemporary Māori orator. Here are extracts from Ross Himona's (2011) narration of the genealogy of the cosmos from the ancient deep unrelenting darkness as it unfurls towards to the vibrant diversity of contemporary life:

Ko Te Kore (the void, energy, nothingness, potential)
Te Kore-te-whiwhia (the void in which nothing is possessed)

Te Kore-te-rawea (the void in which nothing is felt)
Te Kore-i-ai (the void with nothing in union)
Te Kore-te-wiwia (the space without boundaries)
Na Te Kore Te Po (from the void the night)
Te Po-nui (the great night)
Te Po-roa (the long night)
Te Po-uriuri (the deep night)
Te Po-kerekere (the intense night)
Te Po-tiwhatiwha (the dark night)
Te Po-te-kitea (the night in which nothing is seen)
Te Po-tangotango (the intensely dark night)
Te Po-whawha (the night of feeling)
Te Po-namunamu-ki-taiao (the night of seeking the passage to the world)
Te Po-tahuri-atu (the night of restless turning)
Te Po-tahuri-mai-ki-taiao (the night of turning towards the revealed world)
Ki te Whai-ao (to the glimmer of dawn)
Ki te Ao-marama (to the bright light of day)
Tihei mauri-ora (there is life).

Recited in Māori language (a recording is available via a link in Himona's website) or in translation, the repetitions of 'Te Kore'/'the void' and 'Te Po'/'the night' structure this sensual epic of evolution. But the senses here are not primarily those 'five senses' of smell, taste, sight, hearing and touch – at least, not until near the end when, after much restlessness, there is a glimmer of dawn and a sudden burst into the bright day. (In some tellings the dawn takes longer to narrate.) Anticipating future volumes in this series, and the expansion of the idea of 'senses' to include other (sometimes more metaphorical) mechanisms through which knowledge about the world might be gained and integrated, other senses are involved here. There is a sense of longing and anticipation for the 'five senses' to meet the sensual world which is one of feeling, sight and union. As the genealogy continues (see Tawhai 1988), awareness of expansion and growth are replaced by senses of intimacy between Papatūānuku (Mother-Earth) and Ranginui (Father-Sky) and by senses of confinement, frustration and resistance among their first children. This evolves into conflict over desires to separate the parents and then into senses of relief, sorrow, outrage and anger as the great progenitors are separated. Structuring the whole recitation is the expansion of senses of place. It is this sense of place which is vital and generative for Māori speech-makers as they employ narratives like this in creating space for guests and for the new possibilities and responsibilities arising from such relationships.

Introduction

WHAT DOES RELIGION TASTE LIKE?

It is an odd question (especially when asked so abruptly!), but once you begin to think about it religion is intimately associated with food. There are festivals and rituals which it is impossible to name without thinking of food: Christmas and turkeys, Easter and eggs, Pesach and matzah, Ramadan and iftar, puja and prasad. Most religions have rules about food or its avoidance, whether permanently or for set periods or fasts. Religious communities are often formed or broken by decisions about who eats what, with whom, and when. Where there are rules, boundaries are being drawn between those who can be trusted and those who cannot, those who are like us and those who are not. Meal times become key supports for the creation, maintenance and development of ways of being religious. They train children and newcomers in accepted ways of doing religion. They construct communities.

One of the purposes of this book is to improve the practice of the study of religions by increasing attention to sensual, bodily, material and performative matters. Despite considerable efforts to emphasise lived and material religion (e.g. Orsi 1985, 2012; Hall 1997; Nye 2000; McGuire 2008; Morgan 2010; Vasquez 2011; Harvey 2013; Plate 2014, 2015), there are still too many books about religion which fail to recognise the importance of the senses, and of physicality or materiality more broadly. Journals like *Material Religion* and *Body and Religion* promise to change everything! Meanwhile, questions about what religion smells, looks, sounds and feels like in lived reality will be as important as the one about taste in the chapters and books which follow. But, for now, it is the taste of religion – and the sense that we have not yet fully appreciated its religious importance – which we attend to here.

Vasudha Narayanan tells us that

> Several years ago, when I first came as a graduate student to the Center for the Study of World Religions at Harvard University, a fellow student down the corridor kindly loaned me a few introductory textbooks on the Hindu tradition. I read them with considerable interest, and when I returned them, he asked me what I thought of them. With some hesitation – this was my first week at Harvard – I replied that none of them discussed some important features of the tradition.
>
> When asked to expand, I said the first thing that came to my mind: 'Food,' I said and continued, 'my grandmother always made the right kind of lentils for our festivals. The auspicious kind. We make certain vegetables and lentils for happy and celebratory holy days and others for the inauspicious

ceremonies like ancestral rites and death rituals. And none of the books mentioned auspicious and inauspicious times.' (Narayanan 2000: 761–762)

Perhaps it is no surprise that 'lentils' are rarely if ever included in the indexes of scholarly books. However, a quick check of some recent books on key terms in the study of contemporary religions and cultures suggests that 'auspiciousness' also goes unnoticed and under-theorised. Food and the rites of auspicious times deserve to serve as more than colourful vignettes with which to introduce discussions. They can tell us vast amounts about the structuring of families, communities, times and cosmologies. Studies of classical and ancient religious practices and texts (e.g. those related to Vedic and Roman divination) indicate some rich possibilities here.

Piety is, perhaps, more commonly discussed than auspiciousness. However, in their discussion of the geography and morality of Shi'ite Muslims in South Beirut, Lara Deeb and Mona Harb demonstrate the value of linking piety and religious observance with taste in our studies:

> So what makes a cafe legitimate, conservative, or appropriate? There is little consensus on this question beyond the absence of alcohol and non-halal meat. Everyone ranging from religious authorities to devout Muslims to nonpious residents of Dahiya agrees on those two tenets, although few people actually remember the rule about meat unless they are reminded of it, which may also indicate that issues of halal versus nonhalal meat are taken for granted by many in ways that the absence of alcohol is not. Another essential element is the behavior of customers, but here again, where the lines are drawn varies widely, including among the pious. Most pious people agree that such cafes should not play loud music conducive to dancing nor tolerate overt physical contact between unrelated men and women, though again, which music is acceptable and how much physical contact is unacceptable are up for debate. More broadly, there is little agreement on what kind of behavior is appropriate, how people should dress, and where lines of absolute violation occur. Some of these moral boundaries are gendered, though not as strictly as they seem to be in contexts like Cairo. (Deeb and Harb 2013: 7–8)

The 'taken-for-granted' nature of food ways and other matters of taste and consumption (including costume and contact between genders) rewards attention. So too does the question, implicit here but considered more fully in Deeb and Harb's book, of how the sensuality of particular cafes shapes the choices made by people seeking to use their leisure time.

In short, the interactions of taste, sound, touch, sight and smell are all significant in these Shi'ite and other religious ways of negotiating piety.

Perhaps reading novels and other creative narratives would provide us (students of religion) with a better sense of the doing of religion, of religion's roles in people's lives, and of the real causes of affiliation with traditions. Here, for example, are the thoughts of the eponymous lead character of *Life of Pi* on the subject of being Hindu:

> I am a Hindu because of sculptured cones of red kumkum powder and baskets of yellow turmeric nuggets, because of garlands of flowers and pieces of broken coconut, because of the clanging of bells to announce one's arrival to God, because of the whine of the reedy nadaswaram and the beating of drums, because of the patter of bare feet against stone floors down dark corridors pierced by shafts of sunlight, because of the arati lamps circling in the darkness, because of bhajans being sweetly sung, because of elephants standing around to bless, because of colourful murals telling colourful stories. (Martel 2002: 67)

Rather than proliferating the examples here, it is time to outline the structure and contents of this book.

FIVE SENSES TO START WITH

The senses of smell, taste, sight, hearing and touch seemed like a good focus for this first book in a series on religion and the senses. Later books will allow for some challenging additions to the list of possible senses. The idea that religions are deeply and profoundly sensual may be enough to deal with now. Hence, in this book we consider the smells, tastes, sights, sounds and tactile feelings of selected religions. These provide examples rather than an exhaustive coverage. What is true in one religion may prove true elsewhere, or it may provide such dramatic contrasts that we have to wonder how communities and practices could be so different. That is to say, even while focusing on a specific religion in a specific place and time, the following chapters invite and reward considerable comparison.

This book has ten main chapters, two for each of those senses. The first of each set of paired chapters concerns a classical or ancient religious complex; the second is about contemporary phenomena. The study of ancient religions requires attention to material and textual evidence and is increasingly concerned with honing and testing imagination of how people engaged sensually with temples, shrines, healers, statues, sacrificial and votive offerings, processional ways, costumes, meals, and much more. More significantly for our current project, Classical Studies colleagues are providing considerable impetus to what seems to be an emerging multi-disciplinary "sensual turn" to match or rival scholarly interest in embodiment, performance and materiality (see, for example, Routledge's series "The Senses in Antiquity" which dedicates a volume to each of the five senses but also, in Butler and Purves 2013, to synaesthesia; also see Toner 2016 and Betts 2017). The study of contemporary religion can utilise texts, temples, clothes and other material evidence but it also benefits from the opportunity to interview, observe and participate with those who practise and live religions today. Key to our understanding of the study of religions is that there are gaps in our knowledge and that expertise gained in one domain (e.g. in reading ancient texts or in walking with contemporary pilgrims) generates questions and requires ongoing discussion. There are other ways in which this book could have been organised. Later books will not necessarily include chapters pairing ancient and contemporary case studies but they will certainly exemplify and engage with the diversity and dynamism of sensual religion.

The authors of all the chapters have been invited to engage with each other's drafts so that interesting cross-fertilisations could occur. This is particularly true for those paired under the heading of a particular sense. They have also been encouraged to think about the ways in which the sense allocated to them works with the rest of the sensorium (especially but not only with reference to the 'five senses'). The resulting chapters provide pointers to significant literature concerned both with the senses and with the 'case study' material of interest to them. We anticipate that readers will make more connections between the different discussions as well as seeing more gaps that will initiate further research and debate.

Following this introduction, the first section is devoted to the sense of smell. Its chapters take us to visit temples in ancient Samaria and contemporary China. In both locations, religious practitioners made and/or make offerings to deities and/or ancestors, seek benefits from pious acts or reverence, and hope to return home with improved lives. In each case, in different ways, the sense of smell is vital. First of all, an initial approach to Samaritan and Chinese temples involves smelling what cannot yet be seen or touched: the smoke of sacrificial fires and of incense perfumes the air. In the case of the Samaritan temple, devotees are likely to increase this olfactory sensuality by bringing animals for slaughter and cooking. In China, devotees may purchase and light more sticks of incense. Attending to such matters, both chapters enrich our understanding of the sensual doing of religion in specific locations. However, they also present a shared understanding that deities as well as humans associate religious practice or devotion with smells. The deities of Samaria and China smell what is offered to them, and their pleasure in doing so results in them acting favourably towards their devotees.

The second section examines taste. The two chapters here entail a dialogue between special events (such as significant rituals) and everyday life. They discuss the tastes of religion in the Roman Empire (particularly at its northwestern and eastern limits) and in the houses dedicated to the Brazilian religion Candomblé. There are both continuities and differences between meals shared with deities and devotees and those eaten at home, on the street or in more everyday contexts. The authors discuss a rich palette of specific foods enjoyed and sometimes required by particular deities as well as the effects on religious practitioners of regular exposure to such foods. The means of production and facts about disposal are at least touched upon. Not for the first time, these chapters attend to the diversity of religious practice sometimes masked by the use of single words or phrases (such as 'Roman religion' or 'Candomblé') for fluid phenomena.

The third section, about sight, concerns ways in which Byzantine Christians and contemporary Sikhs 'see' deities who are without form or shape. Both traditions have developed material and performance cultures which act as technologies that enable people to 'move beyond what meets the eye'. These chapters challenge us to 'see' sight differently from the common expectation that it permits an immediacy of encounter and relationship. Instead, Orthodox Christians and Sikhs place sight firmly within a multisensory discipline in which visual, auditory and other stimuli work closely together. Although they cannot convey the totality of the divine, it is taught that, treated carefully, such stimuli can serve as the means of coming into the presence (seeing and being seen) of the divine. The paradox is that a strong emphasis on the inadequacy of sight has not diminished the visually stimulating cultures of these Christian and Sikh communities.

The fourth section concerns hearing. It attends to the sounds of religiously and culturally significant events among ancient Greeks seeking initiation at Eleusis and contemporary First Nation and Métis musicians in Canada. An interplay between intensely personal and dramatically communal experiences is just one of the dynamics involved in both discussions. There is also the interplay between structure and improvisation as initiates and musicians expand on traditions of practice, making contemporary and present what has been passed to them to maintain and develop. Interestingly, while those immersed in the 'soundscapes' of these two distinct religious contexts seek to gain some sense of what cannot be seen, they also celebrate the limits of hearing. There are things that cannot be spoken, and some things that must not be spoken. Hearing, then, can be a privileged and encouraged sense, but even as it is emphasised it can also be constrained by a sense that sometimes silence achieves more than sound. In the case of both Eleusis and of Indigenous musical events, the interplay between hearing and other senses deserves the attention offered here.

The chapters of the final section bring us to the matter of touch. In classical Greek and Roman sanctuaries and in Catholic Christian churches and shrines, people come into contact with the divine through tactile media. The shock value of such an assertion may be diminished as it follows on after previous chapters in which encounters with putatively transcendent beings are at least partially mediated by physical senses. The two 'touch' chapters involve containers for purificatory liquids, the architecture of religious buildings, the bodies of those seeking health or fecundity, and statues of sacred beings. Devotees entering religious sites might wash themselves but some of them may even be permitted to wash and otherwise touch and be touched by deities in their material forms. As with other, more mundane relationships, such contact might not be a casual matter but one hedged about with rules and regulations. In distinct ways, the two chapters demonstrate that the results of following or ignoring the appropriate etiquette for touching the divine may be dramatically physical.

FINALLY FOR NOW

There is undoubtedly more that could be said about the contents, case studies and arguments of the varied chapters ahead. We anticipate some excellent conversations arising from reflection on our efforts to expand consideration of religion as a fully sensual (if not only sensual) activity. In case it is not clear, what interests us is not only better description of the doing of religion but also better scholarly approaches. These would respond interestingly to Richard Carp's judgement that

> Our willful unconsciousness of the academic body is literally senseless, and depicts a wishful fantasy of panoptical truth, of a *nowhere* where truth is not dependent on embodiment, situation, culture, or psychology. (2001: 99)

REFERENCES

Abram, D. 1996. *The Spell of the Sensuous: Perception and Language in a More-Than-Human World*. New York: Vintage.

Betts, E. (ed.) 2017. *Senses of the Empire: Multisensory Approaches to Roman Culture*, London: Routledge.

Butler, S., and Purves, A. (eds) 2013. *Synaesthesia and the Ancient Senses*. Durham: Acumen.

Carp, R. M. 2001. 'Integrative Praxes: Learning from Multiple Knowledge Formations', *Issues in Integrative Studies* 19: 71–121.

Christenson, A. J. 2007. *Popol Vuh: Sacred Book of the Quiché Maya People* (Translation and Commentary), online version of original 2003 publication,
URL: www.mesoweb.com/publications/Christenson/PopolVuh.pdf (accessed 3 March 2017).

Deeb, L., and Harb, M. 2013. *Leisurely Islam: Negotiating Geography and Morality in Shi'ite South Beirut*. Princeton: Princeton University Press.
https://doi.org/10.1515/9781400848560

Evelyn-White, H. G. 1914. *The Theogony of Hesiod*.
URL: http://www.sacred-texts.com/cla/hesiod/theogony.htm (accessed 12 March 2017).

George, A. 2003. *The Epic of Gilgamesh*. London: Penguin Books.

Hall, D. D. (ed.) 1997. *Lived Religion in America: Toward a History of Practice*. Princeton: Princeton University Press.

Harvey, G. 2013. *Food, Sex and Strangers: Understanding Religion as Everyday Life*. New York: Routledge.

Himona, R. 2011. 'The Creation', URL: http://maaori.com/whakapapa/creation.htm (accessed 3 March 2017).

King, L. W. 1902. *Enuma Elish: The Seven Tablets of Creation*. London: Luzac.

Lambert, W. G. 2007. 'Mesopotamian Creation Stories' in M. J. Geller and M. Schipper (eds), *Imagining Creation*. Leiden: Brill. pp. 15–59.
https://doi.org/10.1163/ej.9789004157651.i-424.9

Martel, Yaan. 2002. *Life of Pi*. Edinburgh: Canongate.

McGuire, M. B. 2008. *Lived Religion: Faith and Practice in Everyday Life*. Oxford: Oxford University Press. https://doi.org/10.1093/acprof:oso/9780195172621.001.0001

Morgan, D. (ed.). 2010. *Religion and Material Culture: The Matter of Belief*. London: Routledge.

Narayanan, V. 2000. 'Diglossic Hinduism: Liberation and Lentils', *Journal of the American Academy of Religion* 68.4: 761–779. https://doi.org/10.1093/jaarel/68.4.761

Nye, M. 2000. 'Religion, Post-Religionism and Religioning: Religious Studies and Contemporary Cultural Debates', *Method and Theory in the Study of Religion* 12: 447–476. https://doi.org/10.1163/157006800X00300

Orsi, R. A. 1985. *The Madonna of 115th Street: Faith and Community in Italian Harlem*. Yale: Yale University Press.

Orsi, R. A. 2012. 'Afterword: Everyday Religion and the Contemporary World' in S. Schielke and L. Debevec (eds), *Ordinary Lives and Grand Schemes: An Anthropology of Everyday Religion*. Oxford: Berghahn Books. pp. 146–161.

Plate, S. B. 2014. *A History of Religion in 5½ Objects*. Boston: Beacon.
Plate, S. B. (ed.). 2015. *Key Terms in Material Religion*. London: Bloomsbury.
Tawhai, T. P. 1988. 'Maori Religion' in S. Sutherland and P. Clarke (eds), *The World's Religions: The Study of Religion, Traditional and New Religion*. London: Routledge. pp. 96–105.
Toner, Jerry. (ed.) 2016. *A Cultural History of the Senses in Antiquity*. London: Bloomsbury.
Vasquez, M. A. 2011. *More than Belief: A Materialist Theory of Religion*. Oxford: Oxford University Press.

Graham Harvey is Professor of Religious Studies at The Open University, UK. He is series editor for this 'Religion and the Senses' monograph series and co-editor of Equinox's journal *Body and Religion*. His research interests concern the rituals and rhetorics of Indigenous religious and cultural lives.

Section One
SMELL

Chapter 1

A Pleasing Odour for Yahweh: The Smell of Sacrifices on Mount Gerizim and in the Hebrew Bible

ANNE KATRINE DE HEMMER GUDME

On Mount Gerizim, which is close to present-day Nablus on the West Bank, there once stood a temple dedicated to the god Yahweh, whom we also know from the Hebrew Bible. The temple was in use from the Persian to the Hellenistic period (c. 450–110 BCE) and during this time thousands of animals (mostly goats, sheep, pigeons and cows) were slaughtered and burnt on the altar as gifts to Yahweh.

The worshippers who came to the sanctuary – and we know some of them by name because they left inscriptions commemorating their visit to the temple – would probably have experienced an overwhelming combination of sights and sounds and smells: the sight of the sanctuary structure and the imposing views over the valley, the sounds of many people and animals, and then of course the smells – the smell of spicy herbs baked by the sun and carried by the wind, the smell of humans standing close together and the smell of animals, of dung and blood, and as a backdrop to it all the constant scent of the sacrificial smoke that rose to the sky.

In the Hebrew Bible, the temple cult is pervaded by smell. There is the sacred oil laced with spices and aromatics with which the sanctuary and the priests are anointed. Then there is the fragrant and luxurious incense, which is burnt every day in front of Yahweh, and finally there are the sacrifices and offerings that are burnt on the altar as 'gifts of fire' and as 'pleasing odours' to Yahweh. The gifts that are given to Yahweh are explicitly described as pleasing to the deity's sense of smell.

This chapter traces the importance of smell in the sacrificial cults of the ancient Mediterranean, using the temple on Mount Gerizim and the Hebrew Bible as a case study. The material shows that smell was an important factor in delineating sacred space in the ancient world and that the sense of smell was a crucial part of the conceptualisation of the meeting between the human and the divine.

THE PASSOVER SACRIFICE ON MOUNT GERIZIM

It is a spring afternoon on Mount Gerizim near Nablus on the West Bank. Mount Gerizim is a sacred place for the Samaritans, a religious group that lives primarily in Holon in Israel and in Luza on the West Bank and numbers between 700 and 800 people (Magen 2008a: 259–278).[1] As one approaches the mountain a pleasing smell of burning olive wood mingles with the scents of sun-baked earth and herbs that greet the visitor ascending the hill. A crowd has been gathering for hours: the Samaritan men and boys clad in white are in the spacious courtyard, the Samaritan women have gathered nearby and then there are the thousands of tourists that try to see as much as they can of what is going on from the surrounding rooftops and walls. The air is full of smoke from the five fire pits in the ground, which have been stoked with olive wood, and there is a chorus of excited chatter from the crowd and a constant flash from cameras. There is a strong smell of wood smoke in the air and as the night progresses this smell will be supplemented by the enticing aroma of roasting lamb.[2]

According to the Samaritan calendar, it is the fourteenth day of the first month (*Nisan*) and the day of the yearly Passover sacrifice (*Pesach*). At sundown, the high priest begins a prayer and the rest of the congregation

---

1 According to the online newsletter *Samaritan Update*, the Samaritan community numbered 777 people on 1 January 2015 (http://shomron0.tripod.com/TheSamaritanUpdateIndex.htm, accessed on 11 October 2016).

2 I am grateful to Naomi Zeveloff and Dr Ori Orhof for sharing their memories of the Passover sacrifice on Mount Gerizim with me. According to Ori Orhof, the smell of Passover on Mount Gerizim can be divided into three phases: In the late afternoon the pleasant smell of burning olive wood is predominant. In the early evening the significantly less pleasant smells of fresh blood, dung and offal take over, and in the late evening these are supplanted by the mouth-watering smell of spit roasted lamb. For recent 'eyewitness accounts', see Zeveloff (2015) and Lazaroff (2016).

joins in. A long ditch has been dug in the courtyard and along the sides of the ditch dozens of sheep are being held down. It takes two or three men to hold one sheep. At an agreed signal, the men in charge of holding the heads cut the sheeps' throats with large sharp knives and the blood spatters on their white sleeves and trousers and rubber boots. Strong smells of fresh blood and freshly butchered meat and offal begin to intermingle with the pervading smell of wood smoke. The crowd starts cheering and clapping and some of the men proceed to skin and clean the slaughtered animals. Others dip their fingers in the blood and dab it onto the foreheads of themselves and others. Their actions are inspired by the story of the flight from Egypt, which is written in the Book of Exodus in the Hebrew Bible. The Samaritans consider themselves to be the true Israelites, descendants from the northern tribes of the people of Israel. Their religion shares many traits with Judaism, but unlike Jews they only recognise the five books of Moses as sacred scripture, Gerizim and not Jerusalem is their sacred place (cf. John 4) and they have their own ritual calendar (Magen 2008a: 259–278; Pummer 2016a: 9–25 and 195–301).

The fat and the intestines from the sheep are rinsed with water and then they are salted and burnt on the altar, a large metal grid which is placed over a fire at the end of the long ditch. This is the part of the sacrifice that is given to the deity by burning it on the altar (Figure 1.1). The carcass is salted and skewered on a long cooking pole, which is placed in one of the fire pits (Figure 1.2). There is room for about ten sheep in each pit. The fire pits are covered with tarp and a mixture of soil and water is shovelled on top. It takes between two and three hours to cook the sheep in the pits. Around midnight, the pits are uncovered and the whole-roasted sheep are divided between the families, who each eat their share of the meat in haste and accompanied by unleavened bread and bitter herbs. A delicious smell of roasted lamb now envelops the courtyard and wafts upwards in the direction of the many onlookers who can savour the smell but are prohibited from taking part in the meal. As the night draws to a close, any leftovers from the meal are burnt on the altar before dawn (Magen 2008a: 273–278; Pummer 2016a: 260–263; Lazaroff 2016).

The present-day Samaritan Passover ritual combines the prescriptions for the Passover in the Book of Exodus with the rules regarding the 'sacrifice of well-being' (or 'meal sacrifice') in the Book of Leviticus. The Passover ritual in Exodus 12 is not strictly speaking a sacrifice, but a commemorative meal that celebrates the (mythical) story of the release of the people of Israel from Egyptian slavery. No part of the animal is given over to the

22   *Sensual Religion*

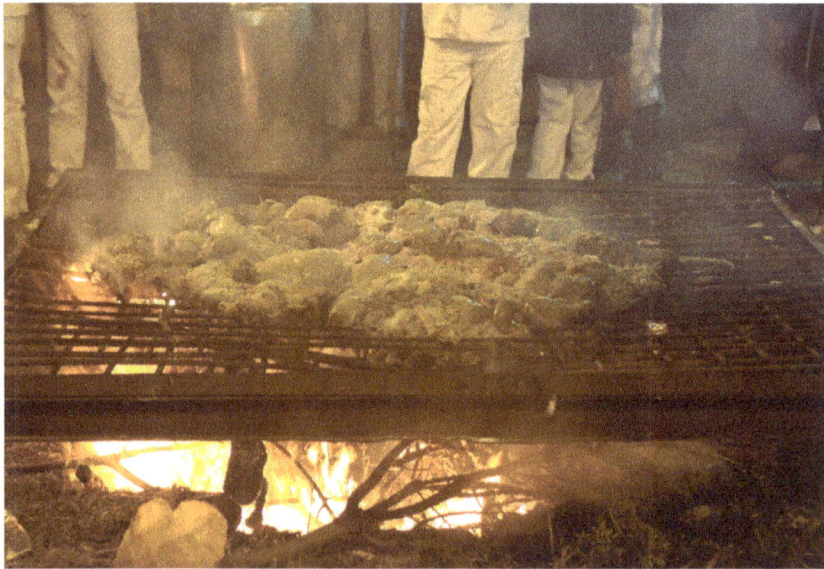

Figure 1.1 Passover sacrifice on Mount Gerizim. The fat and the intestines from the sheep are rinsed with water and burnt on the altar. Photograph generously provided by Dr Ori Orhof.

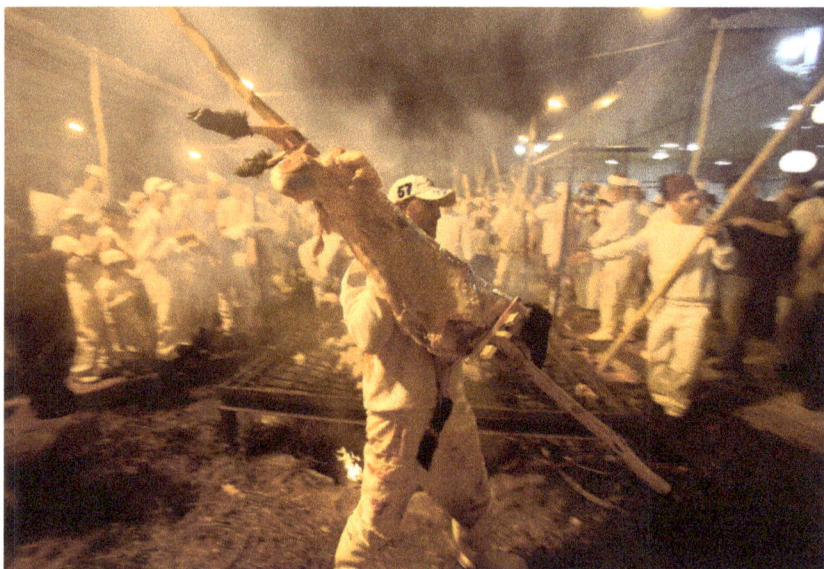

Figure 1.2 Passover sacrifice on Mount Gerizim. The butchered sheep are skewered on long poles and are now ready to be lowered into the roasting pit. Photograph generously provided by Dr Ori Orhof.

deity, the slaughter is profane and performed by laymen, and the setting is the home rather than a temple. It is a meal of whole-roasted lamb that is to be eaten in the home in haste and wearing travelling clothes in order to indicate the urgency of the occasion. In the narrative in Exodus 12, the slaughtering of the lamb also works as an apotropaic ritual intended to ward off the murderous deity Yahweh, who passes through Egypt to kill its firstborns on Passover night, but who 'passes over' (פסח, *pasāḥ*) those Israelite households where the lintels have been marked with the blood of the slaughtered lambs (cf. Eberhart 2002: 274–278; 2011: 30). The sacrificial component comes from the prescriptions for the sacrifice of well-being (זבח שלמים, *zebaḥ šĕlāmîm*) in Leviticus 3 and 7. The special characteristic of this particular type of sacrifice is that it is exactly a *meal*, where the majority of the sacrificial animal is eaten by the donor and his household. The animal's fat and entrails are burnt on the altar as a gift, 'a pleasing odour' (ריח ניחח, *rêaḥ nîḥōaḥ*), for Yahweh (3:5). This division of the animal into the deity's portion and humanity's portion is quite similar to the ancient Greek sacrificial type, the *thusia* (Vernant 1989; Milgrom 1991: 217–225; Jensen 2000: 221–234; Eberhart 2002: 89–111). The sacrifice is performed by a priest in a sanctuary and unlike the Passover ritual, which is a calendrical ritual, the sacrifice of well-being can be performed any time. The Samaritan version of Passover fuses the commemorative meal with the sacrificial meal and as such it maintains a cultic setting for the Passover ritual. This is markedly different from the Jewish Passover Seder, which is a commemorative meal performed in a domestic setting (Pummer 2016a: 260).[3] The Samaritan Passover celebration consists of three elements; it begins with the sacrifice on the evening of the fourteenth day of the first month, which is followed by the seven-day Feast of Unleavened Bread (*Matzot*, cf. Exodus 12:15). On the twenty-first day of the month, the celebration concludes with a pilgrimage to the top of the mountain, where the Samaritan men, again dressed in white, walk in procession before

---

3   The relationship between Passover as a domestic ritual (Exodus 12) and as one of the three annual pilgrimages to the temple in the Hebrew Bible (Leviticus 23:5; Numbers 9:2–5, 28:16; Deut 16:1–6) is not entirely clear. It may simply be a reflection of an inner narrative logic in the text, where the first Passover in Egypt is celebrated in a temple-less age (before the revelation on Mount Sinai) and therefore necessarily takes place in the home, but it may also reflect a historical development of the Passover ritual. For a discussion, see De Vaux (1997 [1961]: 484–492) and Jensen (2000: 215–222).

sunrise to pray and greet the sun on the mountain (Magen 2008a: 273–276; Pummer 2016a: 260–263).[4]

THE SANCTUARY ON MOUNT GERIZIM

According to Samaritan tradition, the Passover has been performed on Mount Gerizim since biblical times. It was on Gerizim that Joshua built his altar when he first entered the promised land (cf. Deuteronomy 27:4-5; Joshua 4:5.20-21), and it was on Gerizim that a number of significant events took place, such as Abraham's near-sacrifice of Isaac (cf. Genesis 22). The Samaritans identify a structure on the mountain known as 'the twelve stones' as Joshua's altar and although they believe that the cult of Yahweh has been carried out here since the time of Joshua they are also adamant that no temple building has ever stood on the mountain. In Samaritan tradition, the cult on Gerizim has only ever been performed as an open-air cult (Magen 2008a: 263–264 and 276–278; Pummer 2016a: 9–13 and 260–261; Pummer 2016b). Whether an actual temple *building* ever stood on the mountain remains a moot point, but recent archaeological excavations have shown that from the mid-fifth century to the late second century BCE there was a thriving sanctuary on Mount Gerizim dedicated to the deity Yahweh (Magen 2008b: 97–180; Gudme 2013: 64–70; Pummer 2016a: 74–91).[5]

The sanctuary on Mount Gerizim was constructed during the Persian period around 450 BCE. In its first building phase the sacred precinct was a relatively small square enclosure (c. 100 × 100 metres) with two main gates in the north and south walls and a few auxiliary buildings.[6] During the Hellenistic period around 200 BCE the sanctuary area was significantly

---

4 The pilgrimage to the mountain to mark the end of Passover is one of three annual pilgrimages in the Samaritan calendar (cf. e.g. Leviticus 23:5). The others are the Festival of Weeks (*Shavuot*) and the Festival of Booths (*Sukkot*). During these pilgrimages, the Samaritans pray at different 'stations' on the mountain, such as the 'twelve stones' (see below). For a good Samaritan resource on these and other festivals, go to http://www.the-samaritans.com/.

5 The majority of the dedicatory inscriptions refer to the deity on Mount Gerizim as 'the god in this place', but one inscription (no. 383) mentions Yahweh by name (Magen 2008b: 235–236).

6 In his reconstruction of the Persian-period precinct, Yitzhak Magen proposes a third gate in the eastern wall (2008b: 103–137), but see the discussion in Gudme (2013: 65–67; and 2015 [in Danish]).

expanded, especially to the south and east, and a number of auxiliary rooms, courtyards and even a fortification were added to the enclosure. In the sanctuary's eastern wall, a third gate was added with a monumental ramp or staircase leading up to it (Magen 2008b: 97-137; Gudme 2013: 64-70; Gudme 2015; Pummer 2016a: 74-91). Also in the Hellenistic period, in the late fourth century BCE, a city was founded just south of the sacred precinct and it grew steadily until it reached a size of about 40 hectares and a population size of up to ten thousand people in the second century BCE (Magen 2008b: 3-93).

The Yahweh sanctuary on Mount Gerizim appears to have been a happening place in the late-Persian and Hellenistic periods; both the sanctuary and the city expanded and a number of pilgrims visited the site to give gifts to Yahweh, and people as far away as the Greek island of Delos and the Egyptian island of Elephantine corresponded with and sent offerings to Gerizim.[7] But in 110 BCE both the popular cult place and the bustling city came to a violent end. The Hasmonean ruler in Jerusalem, John Hyrcanus I, destroyed the city and the sanctuary as part of a campaign that continued his predecessors' rather aggressive expansionist strategy, and neither the city nor the sanctuary were rebuilt after this destruction (Magen 2008b: 178-179; Gudme 2013: 55; Pummer 2016a: 88-89).

Partly due to the sanctuary's violent end, and partly due to subsequent building activity and 'stone-robbing' on the site, it is difficult to get a clear picture of what worship was like on Mount Gerizim. Our best clues come from the hundreds of dedicatory inscriptions and vast amounts of ashes and burnt bones that have been discovered on Gerizim. The dedicatory inscriptions are carved on square hewn building stones (ashlars); they are written mostly in Aramaic, but a few of them are in Hebrew; they all seem to date to the sanctuary's second building phase in the Hellenistic period and they consist of relatively brief dedicatory formulae that refer to something that was given (without specifying what is was) and then give the names of the donor and the donor's dependents. In some of the inscriptions, the donor requests a counter-gift of 'good remembrance':

---

7 In the late fifth century BCE, the Judean colony on the island of Elephantine in Egypt famously sent letters both to Samaria/Gerizim and to Jerusalem to solve a matter related to the Yahweh worship on Elephantine, and in the second century a group of self-designated 'Israelites' made inscriptions on Delos that mentioned the fact that they paid offerings to Gerizim (see Pummer 2016a: 92-96; Kratz 2015: 137-147). In spite of these signs of 'international' relations, the majority of personal names and place names in the Gerizim inscriptions reflect a local group of donors (Magen 2008b: 236-240).

that is, to be remembered favourably and to be in good standing with the deity (Magen 2008b: 227–242; Gudme 2013: 70–90). One of the dedicatory inscriptions was found in its original setting in the monumental staircase outside the east wall, but the rest of them were all discovered in secondary contexts. They are carved on similarly hewn building stones so it is possible that they were part of the same structure that once stood inside the sanctuary enclosure. The director of the recent excavations on Gerizim, Yitzhak Magen, suggests that the inscriptions were carved on an inner wall that surrounded a temple building and sacrificial altar more or less in the middle of the sacred precinct, but since neither the building and altar nor the wall have actually been found, this suggestion remains a hypothesis (Magen 2008b: 100, figure 181, and 227–229; Gudme 2015; Pummer 2016b).[8]

However, in the square adjacent to the Hellenistic-period eastern gate a plaster-covered stone altar has been excavated and around it there were large amounts of ashes and burnt animal bones (Magen 2008b: 120–122). Large amounts of what appears to be residue from sacrifices have also been found in other parts of the sanctuary, e.g. in the southwestern corner where the layer of bones and ashes is two metres deep. All in all more than 300,000 bone fragments mostly from sheep and goats, but also from cows and pigeons, have been found on Mount Gerizim. Most of these were mixed with ashes and pottery sherds and many of them showed traces of burning (Magen 2008b: 160–164).

So what would it have been like for the people who came to worship at the sanctuary – for Amram, and Haggai son of Qimi, and Miriam and all the others, who paid either with money or another kind of offering to have an inscription made and put up in the sanctuary (cf. Gudme 2013: 71–76 and 85–90)? They would probably have been a little out of breath because of the climb uphill and they would have been able to feel the breeze coming from the valley, carrying with it a subtle smell of dust and dry vegetation. On busy days, there would have been quite a lot of hustle and bustle and noise from other visitors and temple personnel, but not as much noise as one may think from the sacrificial animals, mostly sheep and goats, who were awaiting their destiny with surprising calm.[9] However, the animals would have produced a strong smell of dung and of stomach contents when they

  8 Magen believes that the structure known as the 'twelve stones' (see above) is in fact the surviving western wall of the sanctuary's adyton or holy of holies (2008b: 110–114), but the evidence seems to me to be too vague to support such a claim.
  9 I owe this observation and several of the following on the sensory experience of blood sacrifice to the excellent fieldwork carried out by Candace Weddle

were butchered and these smells would have overpowered the smells of fresh and stale blood and perhaps even the smell of many bodies – both animal and human – pressed together in one place (Weddle 2013: 144; Bartosiewicz 2003). On quiet days, the smell of stale blood that had seeped into the ground, pavements and walls and coloured them a dark rusty-brown would probably have been noticeable when there were no other strong smells to overpower it (cf. Weddle 2013: 154–155). We do not know exactly how the sacrifices on Mount Gerizim were performed, but it is not unlikely that some of them were conducted as meal sacrifices where parts of the animal were burnt on the altar and parts were eaten by the worshippers and the priests.[10] Unlike the Passover sacrifice described above, the ordinary method of cooking meat would probably not have been roasting, but rather boiling it in a pot (MacDonald 2008: 32; Jensen 2000: 223–224). There may have been a joyous and expectant atmosphere at the thought of a meal in good company and there may have been an appetising smell of wood smoke and the smell of meat stew and broth wafting up from a number of cooking pots around the sanctuary's courtyards. Behind all of these sensory impacts and smells there would have been a permeating backdrop of scent, namely the constant smell of sacrificial smoke, of burnt bone and fat and flesh, a smell of roasting and charring, which would have risen towards the sky.

A PLEASING ODOUR FOR YAHWEH

In the Hebrew Bible, the importance of the smoke and the smell from the sacrifices burning on the altar is emphasised. The sacrifices are described

---

(2013) in Istanbul during the Islamic Kurban Bayram sacrifices. Subsequently I have watched a handful of recordings of the Passover sacrifice on Mount Gerizim and they seem to confirm Weddle's observations. The sheep remain calm and quiet in spite of the general commotion and even when they are pinned to the ground to be slaughtered they squirm only a little and they do not bleat. See for instance these videos uploaded to Youtube by Tyler Gathro ('Unleavened Bread', https://www.youtube.com/watch?v=nKHF0qEMVVY) and Roger Toye ('Samaritan Passover Samaria 2010', https://www.youtube.com/watch?v=KeZnFTVr1BU), accessed on 11 October 2016.

10 Magen assumes that the sacrifices on Gerizim were carried out in accordance with the sacrificial laws in the Hebrew Bible (2008b: 162), but there is really no evidence for this, since no biblical text has been discovered on Gerizim. See Kratz (2015: 174–178) and the discussion below.

as 'fire offerings' and as a 'pleasing odour' for Yahweh (e.g. Leviticus 1:9, 13.17; Eberhart 2002: 40–52; Eberhart 2004). In the Book of Genesis 8:20–22, the effect of the pleasing odour on Yahweh, which is echoed so frequently in the ritual laws in Leviticus, is unfolded in a narrative about what happens after the great flood. Noah builds an altar and offers sacrifices to Yahweh on it, presumably to thank him for surviving the deluge. When Yahweh smells the pleasing odour, the smoke from the sacrifices, he says to himself that he will never again attempt to destroy the earth and every living creature on it.[11] Yahweh clearly appreciates and enjoys the smell of the sacrifices and he responds to it with goodwill and a promise of protection (cf. Avrahami 2012: 128 and 138; Green 2011: 66–68). There are probably two reasons for this specific emphasis on the smell of sacrifices in the Hebrew Bible; one has to do with Yahweh's particular way of 'eating', the other is related to the fragrant nature of Yahweh's cult. In both cases, the sense of smell is used to make statements about Yahweh's divinity. We shall return to what one could call the Hebrew Bible's olfactory cultic theology below, but first a remark about the relationship between the Hebrew Bible and Mount Gerizim is in order.

The Hebrew Bible is a collection of texts that seem to have emerged from the two Iron Age kingdoms, Israel and Judah, and their Persian-period manifestations, the provinces of Samaria and Yehud. The texts were probably written down during the latter half of the first millennium BCE and although they appear to be recording a *history* that stretches from the creation of the world to the late Persian period, there are many details in the Hebrew Bible's description of events that conflict with so-called extra-biblical evidence such as archaeology and ancient inscriptions. One famous example of this is the goddess Asherah, who is written off as an idol and as the consort of the deity Ba'al by the authors of the Hebrew Bible, but who appears alongside Yahweh as his divine consort in inscriptions from ancient Palestine (Smith 2002: 108–147; Stavrakopoulou 2016; Barton and Stavrakopoulou 2010). In short, the Hebrew Bible is a collection of texts that offer versions of ancient West Asian mythology and history in order to express the authors' ideals about worship and theology. This is true both for the 'historical' and narrative accounts and for the ritual laws, such as the rules for the sacrificial cult in the Book of Leviticus. We cannot assume that these ritual laws describe a cult that was ever practised, but

---

11 The account in Genesis 8 is quite similar to the description of the gods flocking around the smoke of a sacrifice in the Mesopotamian story of Gilgamesh. For a discussion of this and the role of smoke/smell in Mesopotamian sacrifices, see Gudme (2014: 181–183).

they certainly seem to express the authors' vision of an ideal cult, a kind of cultic theology (Grabbe 2003).

There is only an indirect link between the Hebrew Bible and the sanctuary on Mount Gerizim, and that link is the deity Yahweh. Yahweh was worshipped by the people who visited the sanctuary on Gerizim and by the authors of the Hebrew Bible, but there is no indication that the people on Gerizim were familiar with the Hebrew Bible. They may very well have been one of several groups of 'non-biblical' Yahweh-worshippers whose religious world view was not influenced by the Hebrew Bible (cf. the discussion in Kratz 2015: 137–208). Nevertheless, the sanctuary on Mount Gerizim is one of relatively few surviving Yahweh sanctuaries and the Hebrew Bible is by far the most extensive and theologically informative 'yahwistic' text that we have. In this sense, it seems worthwhile to consider – with all the necessary caveats – how the text and the sanctuary may have been informed by one another.

FROM YAHWEH'S DINNER TABLE TO YAHWEH'S NOSE

Let us turn now to Yahweh's special way of 'eating' the sacrifices that are given to him by being turned into smoke on the altar.[12] In the Hebrew Bible, sacrifices for Yahweh are sometimes referred to as the deity's 'food' (לחם, *leḥem*, e.g. Leviticus 21:6; Numbers 28:2) and the altar for burnt offerings is called 'Yahweh's table' (שלחן, *šulḥān*, Ezekiel 41:22, 44:16; Mal 1:7.12). At the same time, the idea that Yahweh simply eats the fat, the intestines and the grain that are burnt for him on the altar does not sit well with the biblical authors.[13] The mental image of Yahweh eating a meal is an anthropomorphism that apparently went too far for the authors of the Hebrew Bible. This is expressed in narrative form in two parallel accounts in the Book of Judges (6 and 13; see also Tobit 12:19), where an angel delivering a message from Yahweh declines an offer of a meal, but converts the meal into a burnt offering instead. The message appears to be that although human beings and divine beings do consume the same foodstuff, e.g. in the case of Judges 6:19 a kid served with bread and broth, they do *not* consume it in the same way. Humans eat with their mouth and divinities eat with their

---

12 For a thorough discussion of this, see Gudme 2014 with references.
13 In the Hebrew Bible, the mouth is connected both with speech and with eating, but Yahweh's mouth is never connected with eating, only to speech, see Avrahami (2012: 124).

noses (cf. Jensen 2000: 291–294; Gudme 2014). This is also expressed in the repeated reference to the sacrifices as 'pleasing odours' for Yahweh. The text stresses that the process of turning Yahweh's portion of the sacrifice into smoke is a necessary condition for Yahweh's acceptance of the gift of food that is being offered to him. Yahweh is ontologically different from human beings and therefore his method of consumption is also fundamentally different from theirs.[14] Yahweh consumes sacrifices through the nose by smelling the pleasing odours that rise from the altar and this is one central aspect of the Hebrew Bible's olfactory cultic theology.

THE FRAGRANT SANCTUARY

Another aspect of the Hebrew Bible's olfactory cultic theology is the general impression of the luxurious and exotic aromas that permeate Yahweh's sanctuary. Apart from the delicious and pleasing odours coming from the sacrifices as they are being burnt, the sanctuary and its priests are scented with the 'sacred anointing-oil' (שמן משחת־קדש, šemen mišḥat qōdeš, Exodus 30:22–33), which is to be applied to both cultic furniture and personnel. Moreover, the anteroom of the sanctuary is enveloped in the aromatic smoke from the incense offerings (קטרת, qĕtōret, Exodus 30:7–9), which are made using Yahweh's own exclusive incense mixture (Exodus 30:34–38).[15] The anointing oil is made of olive oil mixed with myrrh, cinnamon,

---

14 In the case of the sacrifice of well-being, a similar doctrine may be expressed through the different portions allotted to the deity and to the human donors. Inspired by Jean-Pierre Vernant's analysis of the Hesiodic myth of the Greek *thusia*, Hans Jørgen Lundager Jensen has argued convincingly that the sacrifice of well-being in the Hebrew Bible expresses a doctrine about the segregation between the divine and the human realm. The different participants in the meal do share the same animal, but they receive very different portions, and in this difference there seems to be a message about the fundamental ontological difference between god and man (Jensen 2000: 278; Vernant 1989).

15 In Exodus 30, it is stressed how both the sacred anointing oil and the special incense mix is strictly for cultic use and that any kind of profane employment of this oil or incense is forbidden and punishable by death. This prohibition seems to indicate that the biblical authors were familiar with a widespread non-cultic use of spices and precious scents (cf. Jensen 2000: 296–297; Green 2011: 71). Generally in the so-called priestly texts in the Hebrew Bible, it is interesting to see how often incense is involved in narratives that deal with priestly power and privilege (see Green 2011: 77–83).

aromatic cane and cassia, and the objects that are anointed with it become 'most holy', just as the special sacredness of the priests is derived partly from being anointed with this oil (Exodus 30:29; Leviticus 10:7, 21:10-12). Yahweh's incense is made of pure frankincense mixed with stacte, onycha and galbanum.[16] It is described as 'fragrant' or 'sweet-smelling' (סמים, *samîm*) incense and it is to be burnt on the incense altar in front of Yahweh every morning and every evening (Exodus 30:7-8).[17]

Both the incense and the anointing oil mark out Yahweh's cult place as a fragrant sphere and in this way the Hebrew Bible's description of Yahweh's sanctuary corresponds with other ancient West Asian and Greek texts, where both the deities and their temples are said to emanate a lovely smell (Detienne 1977; Nielsen 1986; Reinarz 2014: 25-38). However, the function of the incense offerings in the Hebrew Bible's description of the ideal cult is not entirely clear. Unlike the sacrifices and other offerings that are burnt on the altar, the incense offering is never called a 'pleasing odour' for Yahweh (Green 2011: 72; Eberhart 2002: 309-312). This probably indicates that the incense offering is not thought of as food for Yahweh, but rather serves a different function. It has been suggested that the incense offering is burnt to please the deity and to make him feel at home and comfortable in the sanctuary (Green 2011: 73-77; Houtman 1992; Haran 1960). In addition to this, it may also be that the incense offering serves a double function as it underlines both sacred space and divine presence; just like the anointing oil, the sweet-smelling incense marks the sanctuary as sacred space, as Yahweh's space, and in turn this description of the sanctuary as beautifully fragrant may strengthen the reader's experience of Yahweh's presence. In this way, the luxurious aromas in the sanctuary become both a way of mediating between the divine and human spheres as well as an indication of divine presence on earth (cf. Kenna 2005).

---

16 For Hebrew terms and a discussion of the spices, see Green (2011: 66-71) and Nielsen (1986: 51-67).

17 The incense offering is not the only ritual in the Hebrew Bible in which the use of incense is prescribed. Frankincense must be added to the grain offering before it is burnt on the altar (Leviticus 2) and the offering of the showbread must be accompanied by frankincense as well (Leviticus 24:7). Perhaps most famously, the High Priest is commanded to veil himself in a cloud of fragrant incense when he enters the innermost room of the sanctuary and thereby enters Yahweh's presence on the Day of Atonement (Leviticus 16:12). For a discussion of these other uses of incense in the cult, see Haran (1960); Nielsen (1986: 68-88); Green (2011: 73-77).

THE FRAGRANT ALPHA-MALE

In the Hebrew Bible, there are two particular spheres in which luxurious scents and exotic aromas are described in detail; one is in descriptions of the cult as discussed above and the other is in texts that focus on sexual attraction and seduction, such as the Song of Songs, the Book of Esther and selected passages in the Psalms and the Book of Proverbs (Green 2011: 93–100). This second group of texts make it clear that enticing scents and fragrances are an important component in the construction of sex appeal in the Hebrew Bible. So for instance in the Song of Songs, the female lover is described as a fragrant garden that smells of 'nard and saffron, calamus and cinnamon, with all trees of frankincense, myrrh and aloes, with all chief spices' (4:14). The male lover is also described in terms of scent: 'His cheeks are like beds of spices, yielding fragrance. His lips are lilies, distilling liquid myrrh' (5:13). The sense of smell is very much part of the erotic fantasy in these texts and it is worth noting that the fragrant metaphors are not reserved for women. Although descriptions of women take up more space than descriptions of men (presumably because the texts were written by men), a luscious scent is part of both the masculine and feminine ideal (cf. Reinarz 2014: 114).

In Hebrew Bible scholarship, these two scent-related spheres, the cultic and the erotic, are consistently treated separately, either simply as a means of categorisation (e.g. Nielsen 1986: 68–100; Green 2011: 64–115) or because these two spheres are seen as incompatible (e.g. Jensen 2000: 297–298). However, the Hebrew Bible's non-cultic use of scents may in fact inform our understanding of Yahweh as a fragrant god. The sensual and erotic texts in the Hebrew Bible that stress the allure of sweet smells are also to a large extent texts about royalty and an important part of royal privilege and power in the Hebrew Bible is linked with luxurious spices (Green 2011: 87). A good example of this is King Solomon, who is mentioned several times in the Song of Songs (1:1.5, 3:7.9.11, 8:11–12), and who is presented with spices worth a fortune by the queen of Sheba (1 Kings 10:2.10, 2 Chronicles 9:1.9) and by other foreign rulers (1 Kings 10:25, 2 Chronicles 9:24).[18] In the Book of Esther, the overlap between royalty, sex and scent is parodied in the description of the twelve-month beauty treatment that is

---

18 See also the description of King Hezekiah's riches in 2 Kings 20:13, 2 Chronicles 32:27 and Isaiah 39:2, which includes spices. In 2 Chronicles 16:14, King Asa is buried with spices.

to make Esther and the other virgins fit for a king. It consists of six months bathing in oil of myrrh and six months bathing in spices (2:12).

The symbol of kingship in the Hebrew Bible is to be anointed with (presumably fragrant) oil (e.g. 1 Samuel 10:1). In Psalm 45, a song about a royal wedding, the royal bridegroom is praised as exactly anointed, fragrant, powerful and attractive; the king is 'the most handsome of men' (v.2), his throne 'endures forever' (v.6), his god has anointed him with 'the oil of gladness' (v.7) and his clothes are 'fragrant with myrrh and aloes and cassia' (v. 8). In short, this king embodies the Hebrew Bible's ideal of a powerful male and it just so happens that part of this portrait of privilege and power is to smell good. Considering that Yahweh himself is perceived as a king in some Hebrew Bible texts (Exodus 15:18; 1 Samuel 8:7; Psalm 47:8, 93:1, 96:10, 97:1, 98:6, 99:1 and 146:10) and that kingship was part of the standard 'attire' for ancient West Asian deities (Frankfort 1948; Smith 2002: 91–101), it seems likely that Yahweh's fragrant cult corresponds with his supreme majesty. Therefore I would suggest that we understand the scented symbolism of the Hebrew Bible's description of cult as expressing something about Yahweh as the highest king and alpha-male *as well as* expressing divine presence and divine ontology.[19] Thus, the Hebrew Bible's olfactory cultic theology impresses upon us that Yahweh the king is present in his sanctuary and that he accepts the smoke from the sacrifices as 'pleasing odours' exactly because he is a god.

THE SMELL OF SACRIFICES ON MOUNT GERIZIM

Let us return now to the Yahweh sanctuary on Mount Gerizim in the second century BCE. One of the worshippers who visited the sanctuary was a women called Miriam. She had an inscription made to commemorate a dedication on behalf of herself and her sons. Inscriptions made by female donors are quite rare at Gerizim, but Miriam must have been a woman of independent means, perhaps because she was a widow or a divorcee (inscription no. 17; Magen 2008b: 232–234; Gudme 2013: 75). We do not know where Miriam and her sons came from because Miriam does not include that information in her inscription. Perhaps she thought it was not necessary because everyone including Yahweh knew 'Mother Miriam'.

---

19 Unlike his ancient West Asian colleagues Yahweh does not participate in divine sex in the Hebrew Bible (see the discussion in Smith 2002: 202–207), but this does not mean that he is not cast as a supreme male in many of the texts.

Perhaps she was a thrifty woman who did not want to spend too much money on a long inscription. Only a few of the Gerizim inscriptions mention the donor's hometown, and although the sanctuary on Mount Gerizim did have international connections (see above), these donors come from places close to Gerizim such as Samaria and Shechem (Magen 2008b: 239–241; Gudme 2013: 76). So perhaps Miriam lived close by – she may even have been a resident of the new city that grew up on Mount Gerizim.

When Miriam, who may have been accompanied by her sons and perhaps even by her sons' wives and children, entered the sanctuary she would have been met by a mixture of the smells described at the opening of this chapter: the smell of dung and the stomach contents of sacrificial animals, of wood smoke and meat stew or broth, as well as the smell of smoke arising from the burnt offerings. The smell of sacrifices would have reached the noses of Miriam and her party already when they were ascending the hill on the way to the sanctuary and the smell of smoke and charred and burnt wood and meat would have lingered in their noses and in their hair and clothes after they had returned home.[20] Would the smell of incense and perfumed oil also have been among the aromas that greeted Miriam when she entered the sacred precinct? It seems very likely, based on the frequent use of incense and spices in ancient sanctuaries in general, but since no incense altars or burners and no clear signs of perfume production or use have been discovered on Mount Gerizim we cannot know for sure. And what kind of impression would all of these smells have given Miriam when she came to the sanctuary? If there was even just a partial overlap between the Hebrew Bible's olfactory cultic theology that I have described above and Miriam's thoughts and ideas about what happened at the sanctuary, then we may speculate that Miriam thought of the smell of the sacrificial smoke on Mount Gerizim as a 'pleasing odour' for Yahweh and that this may have indicated to her that Yahweh, the divine king, who eats with his nose, was present there to accept her sacrifices and her gifts and to grant her blessings and divine remembrance in return. In this way, Yahweh's presence in the sanctuary on Mount Gerizim would have been more than just an idea, it would have been a sensory experience, it would have been felt and smelled by Miriam and her contemporaries, and it would have added an ephemeral but still very real sensation of visiting the deity in his home.

20 Again I am grateful to Naomi Zeveloff for her description of how the smell of burning and smoke was difficult to get out of her hair and clothes the next day (private communication).

REFERENCES

Avrahami, Y. 2012. *The Senses of Scripture: Sensory Perception in the Hebrew Bible*. London and New York: T&T Clark.

Barton, J., and Stavrakopoulou, F. (eds) 2010. *Religious Diversity in Ancient Israel and Judah*. London: T&T Clark.

Bartosiewicz, L. 2003. '"There's Something Rotten in the State...": Bad Smells in Antiquity', *European Journal of Archaeology* 6.2: 175-195. https://doi.org/10.1179/eja.2003.6.2.175

De Vaux, R. 1997 [1961]. *Ancient Israel: Its Life and Institutions*. Grand Rapids, MI: Eerdmans.

Detienne, M. 1977. *The Gardens of Adonis: Spices in Greek Mythology*. Hassocks, UK: The Harvester Press.

Eberhart, C. 2002. *Studien zur Bedeutung der Opfer im Alten Testament: Die Signifikanz von Blut- und Verbrennungsriten im kultischen Rahmen*. Neukirchen-Vluyn: Neukirchener Verlag.

Eberhart, C. 2004. 'A Neglected Feature of Sacrifice in the Hebrew Bible: Remarks on the Burning Rite on the Altar', *The Harvard Theological Review* 97.4: 485-493.

Eberhart, C. 2011. 'Sacrifice? Holy Smokes! Reflections on Cult Terminology for Understanding Sacrifice in the Hebrew Bible' in C. Eberhart (ed.), *Ritual and Metaphor: Sacrifice in the Bible*. Atlanta, GA: Society of Biblical Literature. pp. 17-32. https://doi.org/10.1017/S001781600400080X

Frankfort, H. 1948. *Kingship and the Gods: A Study of Ancient Near Eastern Religion as the Integration of Society and Nature*. Chicago: University of Chicago Press.

Grabbe, L. L. 2003. 'The Priests in Leviticus – Is the Medium the Message?' in R. Rendtorff and R.A. Kugler (eds), *The Book of Leviticus: Composition and Reception*. Leiden: Brill. pp. 207-224.

Green, D. 2011. *The Aroma of Righteousness: Scent and Seduction in Rabbinic Life and Literature*. University Park: The Pennsylvania State University Press.

Gudme, A. K. 2013. *Before the God in this Place for Good Remembrance: A Comparative Analysis of the Aramaic Votive Inscriptions from Mount Gerizim*. Berlin: De Gruyter. https://doi.org/10.1515/9783110301878

Gudme, A. K. 2014. '"If I were hungry, I would not tell you" (Ps 50,12): Perspectives on the Care and Feeding of the Gods in the Hebrew Bible', *Scandinavian Journal of the Old Testament* 28.2: 172-184. https://doi.org/10.1080/09018328.2014.932559

Gudme, A. K. 2015. 'Blev templet på Garizim bygget med templet i Jerusalem som forbillede?', *Dansk Teologisk Tidsskrift* 78.3: 261-281.

Haran, M. 1960. 'The Uses of Incense in the Ancient Israelite Ritual', *Vetus Testamentum* 10.2: 113-129. https://doi.org/10.2307/1516131

Houtman, C. 1992. 'On the Function of the Holy Incense (Exodus XXX 34-8) and the Sacred Anointing Oil (Exodus XXX 22-33)', *Vetus Testamentum* 42.4: 458-465. https://doi.org/10.1163/15685330-042-04-03

Jensen, H. J. L. 2000. *Den fortærende ild: Strukturelle analyser af narrative og rituelle tekster i Det Gamle Testamente*. Aarhus: Aarhus Universitetsforlag.

Kenna, M. E. 2005. 'Why Does Incense Smell Religious?: Greek Orthodoxy and the Anthropology of Smell', *Journal of Mediterranean Studies* 15.1: 1-20.

Kratz, R. G. 2015. *Historical and Biblical Israel: The History, Tradition, and Archives of Israel and Judah*. Oxford: Oxford University Press.
https://doi.org/10.1093/acprof:oso/9780198728771.001.0001

Lazaroff, T. 2016. 'In Pictures: Samaritans Perform Sacrificial Passover Ritual', *The Jerusalem Post*, 22 April 2016, http://www.jpost.com/Israel-News/Samaritans-perform-sacrificial-Passover-ritual-452001 (accessed on 11 October 2016).

MacDonald, N. 2008. *What Did the Ancient Israelites Eat? Diet in Biblical Times*. Grand Rapids, MI: Eerdmans.

Magen, Y. 2008a. *The Samaritans and the Good Samaritan*. Jerusalem: Israel Antiquities Authority.

Magen, Y. 2008b. *Mount Gerizim Excavations Volume II: A Temple City*. Jerusalem: Israel Antiquities Authority.

Milgrom, J. 1991. *Leviticus 1–16. A New Translation with Introduction and Commentary*. New York: Doubleday.

Nielsen, K. 1986. *Incense in Ancient Israel*. Leiden: Brill.
https://doi.org/10.1163/9789004275614

Pummer, R. 2016a. *The Samaritans: A Profile*, Grand Rapids: Eerdmans.

Pummer, R. 2016b. 'Was There an Altar or a Temple in the Sacred Precinct on Mt. Gerizim?' *Journal for the Study of Judaism* 47: 1–21.
https://doi.org/10.1163/15700631-12340451

Reinarz, J. 2014. *Past Scents: Historical Perspectives on Smell*. Champaign: University of Illinois Press.

Smith, M. S. 2002. *The Early History of God: Yahweh and the Other Deities in Ancient Israel* (2nd edn). Grand Rapids, MI: Eerdmans.

Stavrakopoulou, F. 2016. 'The Historical Framework: Biblical and Scholarly Portrayals of the Past' in J. Barton (ed.), *The Hebrew Bible: A Critical Companion*. Princeton and Oxford: Princeton University Press. pp. 24–53.
https://doi.org/10.1515/9781400880584-004

Vernant, J. P. 1989. 'At Man's Table: Hesiod's Foundation Myth of Sacrifice' in M. Detienne and J. P. Vernant (eds), *The Cuisine of Sacrifice among the Greeks*. Chicago: University of Chicago Press. pp. 21–86.

Weddle, C. 2013. 'The Sensory Experience of Blood Sacrifice in the Roman Imperial Cult' in J. Day (ed.), *Making Senses of the Past: Toward a Sensory Archaeology*. Carbondale: Southern Illinois University Press. pp. 137–59.

Zeveloff, N. 2015. 'Samaritans Sacrifice Sheep in "Hardcore" Passover Celebration', Forward.com (3 May 2015), http://forward.com/news/israel/307409/samaritans-sacrifice-sheep-in-hardcore-passover-celebration/ (accessed on 31 October 2016).

Anne Katrine de Hemmer Gudme is Professor with special responsibilities of Hebrew Bible Studies at the University of Copenhagen, Denmark. Her research focuses on cult and ritual in the Hebrew Bible in its ancient Mediterranean contexts and she has published extensively on sacrifices and other gifts to the gods.

Chapter 2

Wafting Incense and Heavenly Foods: The Importance of Smell in Chinese Religion

SHAWN ARTHUR

When first visiting Paris' Notre Dame or New York's St John's Cathedral, our vision immediately beholds the grandeur of the architecture and the aesthetics of the space. However, when visiting religious sites around China, our sense of vision may not dominate in the same way. Yes, the gate is beautiful, as are the grounds and buildings, but the most immediately noticeable impression does not relate to sight, but to a different sense: smell.

When approaching a typical Chinese temple, one can see that the entrance gate building is not imposing, but it has interesting decorations and its name in large gold characters on a black background directly above the main door. It likely has upturned corners on its roof, because designers think this helps to improve the energies of the place. Paying a small admission fee, and entering the temple complex, it is very likely that a visitor will not get a chance to look around before their nose is greeted with the heavy fragrance of sandalwood incense in the air. By this, I mean everywhere in the air. In fact, in nearly every temple that I have visited, I have had much the same experience. Sometimes the incense smoke is enough to billow in the wind, while sometimes there is only a faint hint of fragrance having soaked into the temple walls, but I find the unmistakable aroma of burning incense to be a major attribute that creates a temple's atmosphere and sets it apart from other spaces. More to the point, many of the Chinese people with whom I have spoken also find the smell of incense to be the first thing that they notice upon entering a Daoist or Buddhist or folk religion temple – whether urban or rural.

While observing activities in temple settings, I quickly learned that lay people visiting a religious site – be it a temple, shrine or altar – generally perform one central activity as they approach a deity, a Buddha, a divinised cultural hero or their ancestor tablet: they light incense and bow or prostrate themselves (Figure 2.1). Then, people are expected to put a little bit of money in the donation box. Jesuit missionaries called this 'worship,' but the Chinese name for this practice is *shāoxiāng bàishén* 烧香拜神, literally meaning 'to light incense and prostate oneself in front of the divine,' or (*shāoxiāng bàifó* 烧香拜佛 if in a Buddhist place, since *fó* is the Chinese name for the Buddha). Common Western assumptions about 'worship' do not seem to capture the meaning of the Chinese practice, and they could add some misunderstandings as well. I argue that using the actual meaning of the term is more appropriate and accurate.

In the West, common concepts of 'worship' include some emotional commitment along with devotion to or adoration of the deity. However, in China, ritual actions do not necessitate strong emotional states. The Chinese concept refers only to the physical actions of the person; however, many laypeople have told me that it is important to be respectful while doing this. Respect is a core Chinese virtue, emphasised by Confucius, and still prominent in contemporary China.

After lighting incense, the next act is to bow or prostrate oneself. Prostrating refers to kneeling onto a prayer cushion, bowing the head, and placing the forehead, resting on one's hands, on the cushion or the ground in front of it. Westerners call this 'kowtow' from the Chinese '*kòutóu* 叩头' meaning 'to knock one's head' (on the ground). However, in some parts of the country, such as central China, they do not use the word '*bàishén*', to prostrate, but instead they say *jìngshén* 敬神, literally meaning 'to respect the divine' (Chau 2006: 64). This also happens to be the technical term for ritual actions towards one's ancestors: *jìngzǔ* 敬祖, 'to respect or venerate the ancestors', not to 'worship' them.

Here, I focus on the first part of these practices: the burning of incense. The most recognisable aspect of burning incense relates to one of our senses to which it seems few people pay much attention: our sense of smell. Our other senses of sight, hearing, touch, and taste also are important to the full experience of a Chinese temple, but I focus here on the sense of smell because it is central to understanding a temple or shrine's particular kind of atmosphere. When discussing this issue, many laypeople explain that incense smell is crucial for people to experience the temple as prosperous and effective for answering prayers and needs: because this smell means that people use the temple, and not just as tourists.

When Graham Harvey asked that I write a chapter on smell in Chinese religions, I knew this would be a very interesting project. Some of my research indicates that touch is a prominent sense for Chinese lay practitioners, as they like to touch and rub temple statuary for health and good luck, for example. However, after critical reflection on my ethnographic research in China, I conclude that smell is even more fundamental to a typical religious experience.

As I went to work looking for good reference materials for this study, I quickly realised that this topic is woefully understudied among China Studies scholars. In fact, I found relatively few published pieces that mention smell or things related to smell in Chinese religions. Luckily, I have been asking people about the beautiful aroma of Chinese incense every time I visit China. In this chapter, I explore various smells and their meanings associated with Chinese religions – incense being the primary scent-maker, along with foods and firecrackers. I also examine how these aromas can heighten and shape people's memories and emotions, as well as help to foster 'hot and noisy' social aspects of China's temples and religious festivals.

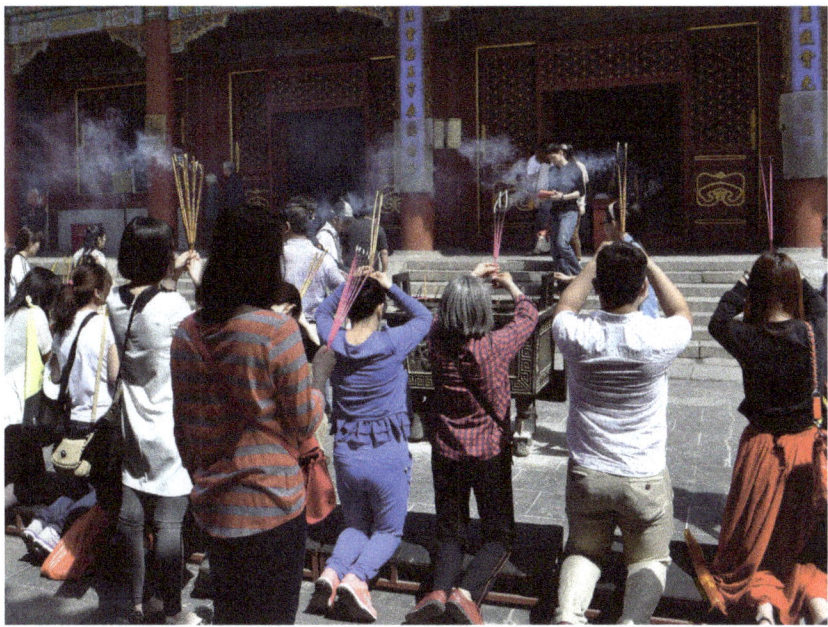

Figure 2.1 The typical Chinese practice of 'lighting incense and prostrating'. Photograph: Shawn Arthur, 2013.

WHAT IS SMELL?

Appealing to some biology and psychology, let us ask, 'What is smell, anyway?' and 'Why might it be important to religionists?' in order to frame our exploration. Smell works when airborne particles enter the nose and get caught on the skin at the back of the nasal passages where there are millions of sensory receptor sites. Humans have about 450 different types of olfactory receptor sites, whereas dogs have 838 by comparison, and it is the combination of signals from these receptors that create what we call smell. The human nose is much more sophisticated than we used to think. Rather than only being able to smell ten thousand different aromas, recent research shows that our noses can distinguish at least one trillion different odours (Henshaw 2014: 28).

Odour particles chemically bind to the proteins in the receptor cells, which then send an electrical impulse along the neurons to the olfactory bulb, at the base of the front of the brain, which begins to process the information (Reinarz 2014: 18). The olfactory bulb is part of the limbic system that deals with emotions and memories – including fight, flight or freeze reactions. The limbic system is one of the evolutionarily oldest parts of the brain (Corbett 2006: 227). The signal also travels to the trigeminal nerve, which can cause physical, facial reactions to smells, such as when our eyes water when slicing an onion (Henshaw 2013: 24).

The limbic system then forwards the scent information to the frontal cortex, where the brain tries to understand and cognitively interpret the aroma signals, and to the thalamus, which sends the information to other neural networks in the brain for connecting to memories, taste and learning (Peace Rhind 2013: 19). Due to the involvement of the limbic system, the major facial nerve and the frontal cortex, we can have strong and immediate emotional, physical and cognitive responses to any smell we experience.

Evidently, we begin to make strong associations between smells and emotional memory from before we are even born (Peace Rhind 2013: 22). Meaning is created from an association of the smell to a particular event or series of similar events – as with the case of lighting incense. Chinese people light a particular type of sandalwood incense to the gods and to the ancestors, but it generally is not used in other areas of life. If people use incense for other reasons, such as to relax in the home, it tends to be of a different type and smell. Making these links between a new scent and one's larger contextual experience can lead to conditioned responses that trigger emotions and memories.

For example, smelling the fragrance of incense each time they enter a religious site within which the person practices reverence, it becomes progressively easy for the person to enter the desired mindset just by getting a whiff of incense smoke. Similarly, having a good experience at a temple festival then becomes ingrained in the psyche through the mechanisms of memory development that are linked to smell. Then, it becomes progressively easy for the person to recall the good feelings, if not the memory itself, when they smell the same aromas or combination of aromas. In this way, smells, emotions, memories and meanings are quite closely linked (see McHugh 2011).

Apparently, even the mere suggestion of scent can affect people's moods and experiences (Henshaw 2013: 38). Following this logic, presenting unlit incense sticks to a deity in circumstances where they cannot be lit could still lead to feelings that the offering is complete and effective. Conditioned responses, perceptions of place, expectations as well as the smell of the unlit incense, all can combine to heighten and shape people's memories and emotions, thus creating very real experiences for practitioners. Additionally, smell can heighten our other senses.

SMELLSCAPES

Imagine, if you will, the scene associated with Adam Yuet Chau's description of visiting a rural community festival.

> The worshiper gets off the bus or tractor-truck, whichever is his means of transportation to get to the temple festival, follows the swarms of other worshipers up and along the valley, passing through noodle stands, watermelon stands, gambling circles, song-and-dance tents, buys a few bundles of incense and spirit money from the incense hawkers, climbs up the steps to the main temple hall, throws the spirit money into the bonfire, lights a string of firecrackers, kneels and prays, burns incense, puts some money in the donation bowl, shakes the divination cylinder and gets his divination slip number, ... goes to the divination slips room and has the divination poem interpreted, then squeezes his way through the crowd to catch a glimpse of the opera performance, and wanders through different parts of the festival ground, snacks or eats a bowl of noodles, chats with acquaintances and co-villagers or complete strangers, plays a few rounds of games, watches the fireworks at night, and always finds himself in the company of tens of thousands of other worshipers .... (2006: 160–162)

Here we encounter many forms of stimuli: strong smells, loud sounds, colourful sights, many tasty foods and people jostling each other for position – all in an environment focused on venerating the main temple deity on its birthday.

It is this atmosphere that is of interest to a few scholars, particularly the aspects that relate to smells. Trying to explain how scent is associated with presence in a place and/or involvement with one's immediate environment, leading scholars call this concept the 'smellscape' (J. Douglas Porteous, cited in Rodaway 2002: 64), the 'aromascape' (Rasmussen 1999: 55), and the 'olfactory geography' (Rodaway 2002: 62; see also Reinarz 2014: 25; Henshaw 2013: 32).

Victoria Henshaw argues, 'Compared with memories gained through other senses, odour experiences can be more frequently recalled after many years, even several decades after they were last experienced' (2013: 31). Thus, the nostalgia produced through scent memories at temple festivals could be very strong indeed and this indicates ways that smell can function in and be influenced by both physiological and sociocultural forces. Kelvin Low advocates that scholars study more of these particular contexts to better understand how 'smells are ordered by and shape cultures ... [as well as] affect and influence our everyday life experiences' (Low 2009: 9).

Yet there is more to this story. The associations that the brain makes are not the only way to influence one's experience through smell. Examining a range of incense ingredients through various medical resources and pharmacopoeia, I found that most of the major ingredients in popular temple incense can function as psychoactive agents, not merely fragrances. As incense is well known to support a meditative state of mind, this might help to explain why incense has positive effects for people, and why temples seem to be sacred and peaceful places.

From archaeological and textual evidence, we know that Daoists from the earliest period, nearly two thousand years ago, used cannabis, calamus (sweet flag) and Sichuan peppercorns in their incense, along with mineral ingredients like lead, cinnabar and arsenic sulphide. Each of these has psychoactive components, which when inhaled in their meditation chambers were likely to produce relaxation and hallucinations (Dannaway 2010: 489–490, 495 n. 9; Avadhani et al., 2013: 601). Similarly, mediums across China are known to inhale hallucinogenic incense smoke in order to facilitate entering a trance state (ter Haar 1999: 7).

Transforming spaces from ordinary to special or even sacred places can happen through use of popular temple incense in China because it contains ingredients such as sandalwood (*tánxiāng* 檀香), which can have a calming effect on the smeller and can act as an anti-aphrodisiac (to assist monks and nuns with maintaining celibacy), and agarwood (*chénxiāng* 沉香; also known as aloeswood), whose smoke has significant sedative qualities (Bazin 2013: 34; Miyoshi et al 2013: 1474; see also Jung 2013). Other important incense materials include musk, ambergris, camphorwood, coarse sawdust, glutinous incense powder, fragrance powders, dye colours and perfume [or essential] oils (Chen 2013: 127; Siripanich, et al. 2014: 138). Thin bamboo sticks are dipped in incense paste, or the paste is hand rolled onto the stick (Chan 1989). Similarly, popular incense in Tibet typically contains a paste of juniper leaves mixed with herbs, saffron, sandalwood, agarwood and musk. Much like sandalwood and agarwood, juniper also has sedative and mind-clearing properties (Bazin 2013: 34), and researchers are finding that even frankincense (*Boswellia* sp.) produces psychoactive effects (Dannaway 2010: 485).

SMELL AS A CULTURAL PHENOMENON

Keeping in mind the biology and psychology of smell with the known characteristics of popular incense ingredients, we can now proceed to discuss how society and culture are integral to understanding the experiences of key Chinese religious smells. Let us start with a little bit of terminology. A common Chinese term for the verb 'to smell' is *wén* 闻, although in ancient China *wén* referred more to hearing or perceiving – since the character contains parts that show an ear pressed in a doorway. The other common term is *xiù* 嗅, which means 'to smell or to sniff'. Chinese has a much richer vocabulary for discussing scents and smells than English, and here are a couple of examples of the way Chinese terms are constructed. *Yòngbíxī* 用鼻吸 means 'to use your nose to breathe', which can infer 'smelling'; *qìwèi* 气味 means 'scent', but the characters mean 'to smell or taste the air'; *xiùjué* 嗅觉 uses the characters meaning 'to smell' and 'to wake up' in order to indicate 'a sense of smell, an atmosphere, or general mood of a situation'.

One thing that creates a good atmosphere is burning incense in a religious site. The term 'incense' derives from the Latin term *incendere*, meaning 'to burn'. This word has a surprising connection to the word 'perfume' as this comes from the Latin *per fumum*, meaning 'through smoke', which seems to indicate a way of communicating with the divine in the Roman context (Rahim 2005: 4418; Moeran 2009: 440). On the other hand, the

Chinese word for incense, *xiāng* 香, means 'fragrance', and it refers to perfumes and aromatic fragrances, especially those made by burning sticks, cones, coils or powders made from a wide range of materials, such as fat and aromatic woods, and using the smoke to attract deities and ancestors (ter Haar 1999: 4–5). The significance of incense to Chinese religions is clear when we look at the large number of words that include the term; for instance, a 'pilgrim' is known as an 'incense guest' *xiāngkè* 香客, 'pilgrimage' is called 'offering incense' *jìnxiāng* 進香, the 'altar' is called an 'incense table' *xiāng'àn* 香案, 'clergy' and 'mediums' are known as 'incense heads' *xiāngtóu* 香头, 'cigarettes' are 'incense smoke/tobacco' *xiāngyān* 香烟, among many others (ter Haar 1999: 5–6).

Additionally, villagers in many traditional and contemporary Chinese communities focus their identities not on the local temple or its main deity, but on the incense-burner (*xiānglú* 香炉) itself, and this is why in southern China, the head of a local social unit is called the 'chief of the [incense-]burner' (*lúzhǔ* 炉主). Among many communities, locals have stories about the incense-burner in their temple – what it originally looked like, how it was destroyed during the Great Leap Forward in the 1950s when almost all spare metal was melted to make steel, and how a couple of families or the volunteer community raised money to commission a new casting. The incense-burner is likely a focal point because the origin of modern incense-burners is in ancient Chinese bronze vessels that held sacrificial foods for the divine, and there are indications that incenses were used back into the Zhou dynasty (1025–256 BCE), long before the arrival of Buddhism in 68 CE (Milburn 2016: 441).

We have discussed that the Chinese word for 'worship' (*shāoxiāng bàishén* 烧香拜神) includes the order to light incense to the gods; and I agree with ter Haar that the burning of incense is the 'truly the most fundamental religious act in Chinese culture' (1999: 5). Yet the Chinese light incense for a wide variety of reasons that have multiple layers of meaning beyond merely respecting deities and spirits.

INCENSE AND SMELL USE IN CHINESE RELIGIONS

We continue with an examination of a typical temple organisation. The main gate is in the south, and the largest buildings, which are shrine halls, are along the central axis towards the north – with each shrine hall getting larger towards the back. This is because many Chinese temples are built to symbolise a sacred mountain. The visitor starts at the bottom of the

The Importance of Smell in Chinese Religion 45

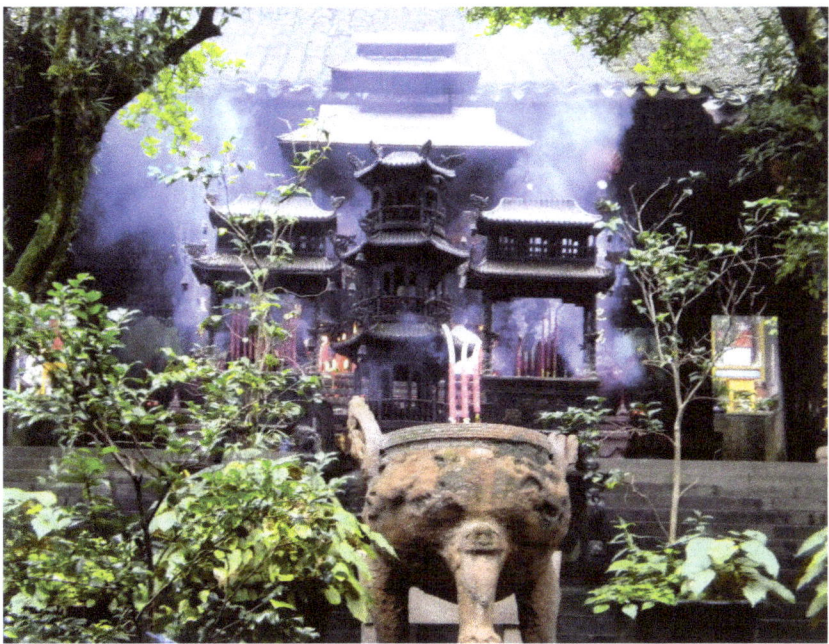

Figure 2.2 Cloud of incense on Mt Qingcheng, Sichuan, China. Photograph: Shawn Arthur, 2013.

mountain and works their way up each peak and valley until they reach the summit, which houses the most important deity statues. These temples also have a variety of natural elements such as foliage, fragrant flowers and trees, which together bring in other mountain elements. Why mountains? Because their peaks are in the clouds (almost like clouds of incense), where immortals live and where one could be physically closer to the gods who live in the heavens (the stars).

Incense assists with the creation of the temple as sacred mountain, and thus the temple as sacred space (Figure 2.2). As soon as visitors cross through the gate house, they usually can begin to smell burning incense or the lingering aroma of years of incense smoke that seeped into the walls. Since it is not noticeable on the sidewalk next to the temple, it is as if the temple walls themselves want to keep the aroma inside.

The clergy who work and/or live in the temple regularly light incense in front of each shrine hall, and visitors who wish to respect the gods will follow suit. In this way, the use of incense – the scent, people's experience of it and its symbolic meaning – helps to demarcate and create the special atmospheres that temples have. Combining all of these layers in their awareness, on a typical day Chinese visitors and pilgrims are able to walk through the entrance gate as if it is a gate leading away from the normal world into a sacred time where stress disappears, traffic and crowd noises are gone, and one is reminded to adopt an attitude of respect, reverence and morality.

Along with the physical setting, temples have explicit and implicit rules for behaviour. In this way, the temple becomes 'sacred' in the Durkheimian sense of 'being set apart and forbidden'. However, on a festival day, the atmosphere changes dramatically to one of noisy and boisterous celebration, and the thick plumes of sandalwood incense contribute positively to the 'hot and noisy' sociality of the event. I address this phenomenon in more detail shortly.

SMELL AND COMMUNICATING WITH GODS, SPIRITS AND ANCESTORS

Following from our theme of incense facilitating sacred space, incense smoke and other fragrant aromas often imply the presence of, or a connection with, the divine, a Buddha or an ancestor. In formal religious rituals, burning incense is the first act, and it is meant to invite the divine to be present during the ritual. Blake and Clements explain one metaphor behind this action in that an aroma is not solid, it is a disembodied phenomenon – much like spirit beings that someone wishes to attract. Ritualists then take for granted that the divine heeds the invitation, and they assume the divine is present (Blake 2011: 91; Clements 2014: 46). In a similar way, Moeran points out that 'the words of the Buddha were said to be fragrant, [and] the smell of incense was thought to invoke the Buddha's presence' (2009: 440). In fact, Christianity calls this idea the 'odour of sanctity', meaning that worshippers know the divine presence due to the noticeable pleasing fragrance (Classen, et al. 1994: 52; Low 2009: 21).

Jonathan Reinarz argues that incense smoke and fragrance were associated with religion from its earliest history because these could be tangibly sensed but not seen, heard or touched (Reinarz 2014: 19). The scent and smoke of the incense or fragrant paper rises to the heavens while people show reverence or pray for assistance. Thus, the burning incense becomes the most common and important mediums for human-divine communication and interaction. Subsequently, the aroma marks this process (Rasmussen 1999: 64; Reinarz 2014: 32; see also Milburn 2016: 442).

INCENSE AS SACRIFICE AND OFFERING

Of what does this communication consist? Typically, people use candles and incense as offerings – along with some money in the *gōngdé* 功德, the so-called 'virtuous action' box – as they ask for assistance or say thanks to the deity for helping them in the past. This process is the key to Chinese religions: maintaining one's relationship with the divine (on behalf of oneself and/or one's family) through respect and reciprocation. Originating in ancient China and becoming essential under Confucian socio-political structures, respectful and reciprocal relationships are still the ideal socio-culturally determined behaviour among humans and between humans and the divine (Jackson 2011: 613).

Practising this ideal model for interacting with the divine begins with burning incense, giving a donation and making a vow (*xǔ yuàn* 许愿) based on what a layperson needs and what they can give. Then, when one's prayers are answered, one is obligated to return to fulfil the vow (*huán yuàn* 还愿) (see Administrator 2009). Whether addressing their prayers to the folk God of Wealth, the Daoist God of Medicine, Confucius the Ancestor of Education, or Guanyin the Buddhist Goddess of Mercy – or all of the above – people use the same model.

Basically, what happens is that the person is setting up a barter contract by giving an offering with the prayer. The person then expects an obligatory reciprocal response from the other-than-human being. In the Chinese world view, deities are alive, present, and have agency – not as a statue, but as a metaphysical 'person,' and one of their jobs is to assist humans with their needs. Therefore, this barter system is not disrespectful at all, it is seen as quite respectful because the person is essentially paying for part of the assistance up front.

Regarding offering incense, not all incense is the same. Incense commonly comes in cones, coils and sticks; but the sticks can be thin and small or huge (Figure 2.3). I mention this because there is one aspect of offering incense that is somewhat controversial among Chinese religionists: using large sticks of incense. The term *shāogāoxiāng* 烧高香 means 'to burn tall incense', and it has the implication of 'thanking profusely'. In many cases, people, especially men, buy and burn a large incense stick in order to demonstrate their seriousness and the importance of their problem or issue. However, as the middle class in China is growing rapidly, and they have extra money, a growing number of younger men seem to be purchasing and burning the largest incense sticks in the temple to show off their new wealth and social stature – and what seems to many older adults to be

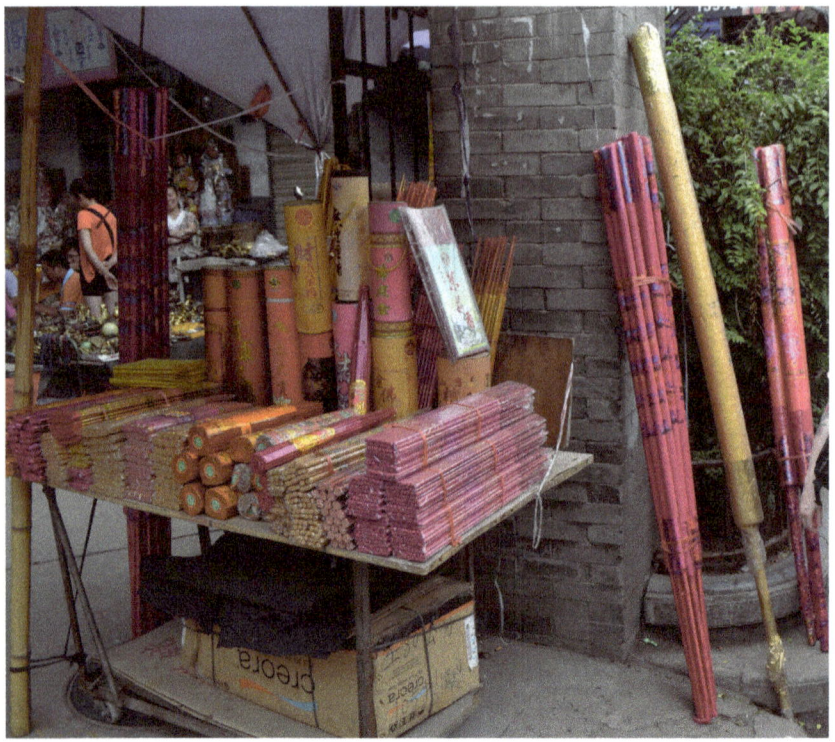

Figure 2.3 Types of incense, Xi'an, China. Photograph: Shawn Arthur, 2013.

an inflated sense of self-worth. In other words, a serious means of asking for help is being co-opted as a status symbol, which many people think is unethical and crass. Of course, without asking the person why they lit a massive stick of incense, no one would know the answer with certainty – it could be to show off or to respectfully pray for family and friends in crisis.

FORMING RELATIONSHIPS THROUGH SCENTS

Beyond respect, the most crucial aspects of human-to-deity relationships are mutual trust (*xiāngxìn* 相信) and reciprocity (*gǎnyìng* 感应). To mutually trust means to trust that the other 'person' will uphold their obligations in a mutually reciprocal and beneficial relationship. Also, the Chinese understanding of 'reciprocity' is strongly linked to concerns about acting appropriately (*lǐ* 礼), cultivating morals and harmonizing one's interpersonal relationships (guānxi 关系) (Feng 2011: 29, 120–121; Yao and Zhao 2010: 10, 197).

Much as with 'worship', Westerners often misinterpret what is happening here by translating 'mutual trust' as 'belief', but the Chinese language does not have a term for the noun 'belief' – as in 'I have a belief' – and they do not think in terms of 'believing in' something. Rather, mutual trust refers to 'believing' that the other party will uphold their end of the bargain.

Here, we can link to similar ideas and practices across the globe. We can use Graham Harvey's concept of 'animism' to think about Chinese perceived relationships with the divine. Harvey defines 'animism' as 'the attempt to live respectfully and reciprocally as members of a diverse, multispecies community of living persons (only some of whom are human) – and all of which deserve respect' (Harvey 2012; 2013: 126). For Harvey, 'persons' – even other-than-human beings – are known to be 'persons' when they interact and communicate with other 'persons' including deities, ancestors and other spirit beings in certain ways – such as respectfully, reciprocally and at least somewhat willingly (Harvey 2013: 124). Similarly, for many Chinese, their practices with incense emphasise 'animistic' reciprocal communication, cooperation and mutual respect – which they experience when venerating their ancestors and the divine (see Yao and Zhao 2010: 40); and people strive to avoid offending any deity or ancestor (see Zavidovskaya 2012: 183).

BURNING INCENSE AS A MEANS OF PURIFICATION, HEALTH AND CLEANLINESS

In addition to external communication, a number of my interlocutors explained that when one lights incense, it shows one's internal character – whether one is doing it 'appropriately', or in other words, following religiously-created and socially-sanctioned norms for bowing properly, showing generosity, being respectful and serious, and the like. Staub et al. interviewed a Buddhist nun who said, 'Burning incense…is a statement of not doing bad things any more. Through the burning of incense, you settle down [and] you get rid of hardness' (2011: 11). Additionally, once the incense is lit, the bows completed and the prayers all said, incense becomes a symbol of the laity ensuring the protection of their health and well-being. Thus, upon smelling incense, their expectations are renewed and reinforced. This brings people to their local temple on Chinese lunar

New Year's Day to 'Burn the First Incense Stick', which people believe will bring them great merit, good fortune and well-being.

While clergy and laypeople use incense to promote health, people also use its smoke to cleanse and purify themselves, places and things. Thinking of Mary Douglas' influential theories about purity and pollution, there are a range of formal rituals across Chinese religions that use incense smoke – with its primary qualities of burning and emitting a sweet aroma – for purification purposes (see Rahim 2005: 4418; Staub, et al. 2011: 7–11). In fact, some of the earliest Chinese written sources indicate that people burned aromatic woods and plants to drive out malignant energies or spirits such as ghosts (ter Haar 1999: 5) – and these types of practices continue today in both official and folk religious traditions. In Chinese temples, to burn incense and to be covered in incense smoke is simultaneously to be purified and ideally to reflect on one's morality in these sacred places.

INCENSE AND RITUAL

It is Chinese ritual tradition to burn incense before and during all formal religious rituals, and many informal ones as well. Different religions have special ways of holding and burning incense, but the goals and the expectations of the laity are quite similar across traditions – respect, communication, purification and such.

Many people burn incense without deity reverence, but in religious connotations, it is common to burn incense in front of an object of veneration, such as at ancestral and kitchen god altars and during meditation practice, but also as people read, or even recite, religious texts and scriptures (ter Haar 1999: 3–5). By the sixth century CE, Chinese monks were even using varying lengths of incense to mark time during meditation and other practices (Rahim 2005: 4419). In 1870, missionary Justus Doolittle wrote:

> The Chinese use an incredible amount of incense yearly. Some families use it daily, others only on set occasions, as on the 1st and 15th of each Chinese month, on birthdays, or when, for any special reason or occasion, they desire to worship the god of the kitchen, or their ancestral tablets, or their household gods generally. In temples, by the priests, large quantities of incense are burned. Before the principal idols incense is kept continually burning. The people, in their occasional or periodical visits to the temples for religious purposes, always burn incense. (1870: 236)

Smell is also important to Daoist and folk religious formal rituals, where candles, incense, food, paper and firecrackers represent the cosmic Five Phases of water, metal, earth, wood and fire, respectively. Each ritual material is meant to heighten the senses, and incense and firecrackers hold special significance as we have discussed (Blake 2011: 83). According to Fred Blake,

> the candles bring forth a flickering glow that makes the cosmos luminous; incense provides a smoldering fragrance that permeates the cosmos with desire for the...presence of spirits; food provides flavorful sustenance, ... and sustains life; paper money shifts the active mode of [awareness] ... from the [taste] of food ... to the touch of paper ..., in making and circulating things of value. [...] And finally, popping firecrackers dispel the residues of solemnity with playfulness (*rènào*). (2011: 86; also see Jochim 1990)

SCENTS OF FOOD AND FIRECRACKERS

Let us move on to examine another significant smell: the aromas of food. We examine food because we know that aromas affect and can complement taste. I am referring not to home-cooked comfort food, but rather to restaurants, volunteers and food-cart vendors present in temples and at temple festivals.

The first smells of food up for discussion relate to temple restaurants. A number of larger temples have restaurants on-site to feed guests. Daoist and Buddhist restaurants are vegetarian because members of both groups have taken vows to avoid killing – and that includes being involved with the killing of animals. These cooks create some of the best-tasting foods on the planet. Using a wide range of vegetables, mushrooms and fungi, tofu (*dòufu* 豆腐) and different starches like root vegetables, they are able to create delicious vegetarian versions of normal meat-based dishes without harm to any sentient being. Sometimes visitors can smell the aromas of freshly cooked food coming from these restaurants, and this creates good connections with the temple – and perhaps the religion as well.

Second, many Buddhist temples sponsor associations of local regularly-visiting laity, and once a month these volunteers prepare a vegetarian meal with noodles and soups for temple-goers that day. This is one way that the laity can generate good merit – by helping the community in need – with free food and free entrance to the temple. Members of these lay associations create a welcoming atmosphere, which includes good conversation, generosity, and tasty, good-smelling foods.

Third, Chinese temples celebrate the birthdays of some of the popular deities whose statue representations are housed inside. These birthday 'celebrations' often involve special foods associated with the deity. For example, Mazu, the 'matron ancestor', who is a Goddess of the Sea, evidently likes vegetarian dumplings and longevity noodles. On her birthday, lay volunteers prepare and serve hundreds of small bowls of these fresh-smelling foods to the large crowds in the temple. Receiving and eating these foods is considered to be very auspicious, as they are supposed to be blessed by the goddess. People even wait in line for these dishes and only eat one dumpling so they can bring the rest home for their families to share, and thus partake in the blessings as well.

Fourth, and last, we have foods associated with large holiday festivals and temple fairs, where delicious smells of food fill the air from a wide range of nearby restaurants and street vendors with their food-carts. Walking through the crowds at one of these events one could encounter nearly any food – from roasted nuts and candied fruit, to fried rice, soups and noodle dishes, to spicy dishes and stinky *dòufu*. The smells can be strong or subtle, but they are a welcome addition to the festivities. The foods are eaten by hand or in small bowls, more as a snack than as a full meal, so people can eat a variety of foods to improve their overall experience of and excitement with walking around at a busy and crowded festival all day.

Adam Chau describes the cacophony of aromas at a large rural festival for the Black Dragon King:

> The smells and tastes of all kinds of food: noodles made of wheat and potato flour, griddle cakes, goat intestine soup, stir-fried dishes, garlic and scallion, vinegar and red pepper, watermelons, small yellow melons, ideas, soft drinks, burning liquor, beer; the pungency of diesel exhaust fumes, firecrackers, freshly slaughtered pigs and goats, and their warm blood; the mixed fragrance and pungency of incense and burning spirit money; the faint smell of sweat from so many people squeezing through the main temple hall. (2006: 160)

The constantly changing yet pungent range of smells here provides a sense of the richness of a rural temple fair atmosphere. Along with these fair foods, festival events ideally have a very celebratory atmosphere with many different activities going on all day and into the night, and this is accentuated by people periodically lighting a string of firecrackers to invite the gods and to scare away negativity.

People light firecrackers at holidays, temple festivals, marriages, funerals, the Chinese lunar New Year, the Qingming grave sweeping day, business openings and other occasions. They may be used to wake up the local Earth God, but they are generally used to rid the area of unwanted energies, ghosts and harmful earthly spirits. At these events, people just light a string of firecrackers, they do not need an elaborate show of fireworks – which would not have the same effect because shooting fireworks make their loud noises high up in the air rather than close to the ground where they are needed to disperse malignant energies. As a result, the aroma of burnt gunpowder mingles with food and incense smells and contributes to the lively atmosphere.

SOCIAL IMPLICATIONS OF INCENSE USE AND SOCIAL MEANINGS OF SMELL IN CHINA

The term for the desired festive atmosphere is *rènào* 热闹, literally 'hot and lively or noisy', and it refers to a social atmosphere that is enjoyable, energetic and exciting. The 'hot' of 'hot and noisy' is made of multiple layers of experience: heat from strung up lights, food vendor stalls, burning candles and smouldering incense sticks. As large numbers of people light and place bundles of incense sticks in the incense-burners to smoke, the incense gives off a slight ambient warmth (especially if the sticks catch fire). The boisterous nature of these events is exactly what organisers and sponsors hope to achieve: a lively spectacle that everyone enjoys and which brings the community closer together for a short time. Whereas *rènào* is the hallmark of a successful festival or celebratory atmosphere, I argue that smell is a central feature in this concept. Without the smells of cooking foods, burning incense, firecracker smoke, cigarette smoke, sweaty people and such, a sense of *rènào* could not be achieved (see Chau 2008: 490).

Of course, the sounds of fireworks also contribute to the 'hot and lively' atmosphere expected at special temple and community events. They are an exciting addition to all the other noises associated with a crowded area of celebrants, tour groups on pilgrimage, food and merchandise vendors trying to capture the attention of each passer-by, music and other local entertainment such as opera troops, formal ritual music with its cymbals, drums and chanting, and so on.

Some incense-burners require people to bend over under a metal canopy to place their incense sticks into the sand and ash. When there are enough people doing this, the bundles of sticks can spontaneously catch on fire causing much excitement and crowds who want to add their bundles to the blazing fiery pile. To avoid too much smoke or spontaneous fires in the incense-burners, some temples will cover the incense-burner and have people just place their unlit incense on the cover or on the altar in front of the deity, since the incense seems mostly to be an offering in the first place, and lighting it is secondary (it is the customary means of presenting the offering). Due to associations of memory, of burning incense and its smell, unlit incense offerings can be equally effective for participants.

Smell is not only important to emotions and senses of place, but also socially, as with the people who take a moment to recognise all of the other people around them who have and are experiencing the same particular circumstances in a temple or large festival setting. This can lead to a sense of collectivity and group cohesion – at least for a short time. To burn incense and prostrate oneself is also to show willingness to participate in socially responsible and 'culturally-constituted behavior[s]' (Jackson 2011: 613) of respect. As Rasmussen argues, offering perfume and incense to others acts as a mark of social personhood and belonging (1999: 63). Here I suggest that we recall Graham Harvey's (2012) idea of animism, and we can see that offering incense to other-than-human spirits and divinities constitutes an attempt to live respectfully in a diverse world. Smell, then, functions as a social marker as well as an aesthetic one.

WHY LIGHT INCENSE?

Why do people go to temples and light incense? The incense packets themselves depict some intended desires that people want. Figure 2.4 shows a selection of incense boxes from different temples. The names of these products are: *Beckon Money*, twice on the left, *Pray for Good Fortune*, and then three different *Peace and Harmony* incenses on the right. Many of the more expensive and larger sticks of incense also have prayers written on the incense, such as a popular yellow stick that says, 'incense for a wealthy and beautiful home and long life'. Most bundles of small, thinner incense have a band around them that says, 'peace and harmony for the whole family'. During busy temple days, on holidays, and full and new moons, people will even go through the garbage and recycling bins at a site to collect these wrappers. Because they are associated with the temple, and they have the blessings written on them, some people see these wrappers as a form of paper that can be burnt as a prayer for their well-being.

Additionally, I have compiled the range of reasons why lay people visit religious sites to light incense and prostrate themselves (see Arthur 2018). People also touch auspicious statues and words in temples and purchase a wide range of charms and talismans to hang in their environment, that are supposed to provide good luck and blessings for them.

The most common issue that surfaced during my research was that people are trying to control life's situations in order to achieve a general sense of well-being, prosperity, harmony and improvement in their lives. In trying to accomplish this goal, people work to attract the influence of other-than-human persons or powers (deities and/or ancestors), and they seek protection, economic security, figuring out their destinies, controlling fate and fortune, and solving personal and home life issues (see Arthur 2018; Arthur and Mair 2017). The well-being that these laity search for includes better ways to deal with and solve the problems that they face in life, looking for hope in bleak circumstances, and working to better understand themselves and why life is the way it is. Over and over people told me they came to a religious site seeking health, safety and peace for themselves and their families.

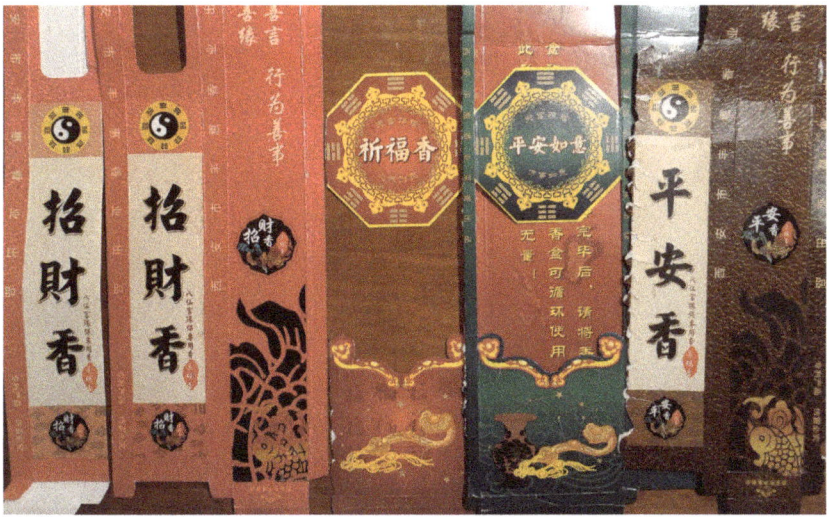

Figure 2.4 A selection of Chinese incense boxes. Photograph: Shawn Arthur, 2013.

NEGATIVE HEALTH EFFECTS OF INCENSE

Our exploration of smell in Chinese religions has thus far focused on positive aspects; however, the fragrant smells of incense can come at a price. Although agarwood and sandalwood have a range of health benefits when ingested (Hashim et al. 2016; Mohagheghzadeh et al. 2006), burning agarwood- and sandalwood-based incenses indoors or everyday can have negative effects on the person inhaling the fragrant smoke. Research shows that incense contains a range of heavy metals and other carcinogens that have been proven to have negative health effects on factory workers who make incense and temple workers who inhale incense smoke throughout each day. As one might imagine, lung and upper respiratory cancers, asthma, leukaemia and contact dermatitis are some of the common diseases stemming from the regular inhalation of incense smoke, especially the heavy smoke associated with temple festivals and holidays (Siripanich et al. 2014: 138; Lap et al. 2011; Seow and Lan 2016: 155; Navasumrit et al. 2008; Chiang and Liao 2006). Lin et al. argue that 'in order to prevent airway disease and other health problem, it is advisable that people should reduce the exposure time when they worship at the temple with heavy incense smokes, and ventilate their house when they burn incense at home' (2008: 1).

CONCLUSION

Looking at the speed at which temples across China are being reconstructed and religious activities are resuming, one might get the impression that Chinese people are very religious. However, survey data and people's responses when interviewed indicate that very few Chinese people admit to being religious. Part of the reason for this is Chinese connotations of the term *zōngjiào* 宗教, which originally meant 'ancestral teachings'. When the new meaning of the term as 'religion' came from Japan in the 1860s, it also came with the connotation of 'the Christian way' of being 'religious' – such as having strong beliefs and faith, being exclusive to one tradition, devotion to a single deity, being antagonistic to other traditions, etc. Given that few Chinese people focus on these things in their lives, it is no wonder that only around ten percent of many survey participants agreed with the statement that they were 'religious.' Even when talking to people in temples just after watching them light incense and prostrate themselves, they would say they were not 'religious' (*zōngjiào*).

However, as researchers become more aware of the Chinese context and ask about venerating ancestors and lighting incense at a temple, the percentage of positive responses grows to over eighty percent. I found this as well in my visits to China. Many Chinese people use the technology of what we call religion – such as charms, talismans, incense, candles, bowing in front of a deity statue and touching auspicious statues – for safety, luck, health and the like. And I find that smell – especially of incense, temple foods and firecrackers when appropriate – plays a key role in people's perceived successes.

The phenomenon of 'religions' in China does not rely on a personal psychological state or an emotional commitment, but the smells in religious spaces can and do elicit these states. As we have seen, the often taken-for-granted sense of smell in religious life also reflects larger social ideals and structures, such as its emphasis on respect, reciprocation and fulfilling mutual obligations. Since incense smoke has been one of the most important ways that people feel they can communicate and interact with the divine and with one's ancestors, we must consider smell when we attempt to understand Chinese religions and culture. In fact, when asked why they light incense, many people told me, 'It's just part of being Chinese!'

REFERENCES

Administrator. 2009. 'Burning Joss Sticks and Worshipping Spirits' in FYSK Daoist Culture Centre Database.
http://en.daoinfo.org/wiki/Burning_Joss_Sticks_and_Worshipping_Spirits (accessed 25 January 2017).

Arthur, S. (2018). *Contemporary Religions in China*. New York: Routledge.

Arthur, S., and Mair, V. 2017. 'East Asian Historical Traditions of Well-Being' in R. J. Estes and J. Sirgy (eds), *The History of Well-Being Throughout the World*. Cham: Springer. pp. 59–82. https://doi.org/10.1007/978-3-319-39101-4_3

Avadhani, M. M. N., Selvaraj, C. I., Rajasekharan, P. E., and Tharachand, C. 2013. 'The Sweetness and Bitterness of Sweet Flag [*Acorus calamus* L.] – A Review', *Research Journal of Pharmaceutical, Biological, and Chemical Sciences* 4.2: 598–610.

Bazin, N. 2013. 'Fragrant Ritual Offerings in the Art of Tibetan Buddhism', *Journal of the Royal Asiatic Society* Series 3, 23.1: 31–38.
https://doi.org/10.1017/S1356186312000697

Blake, C. F. 2011. *Burning Money: The Material Spirit of the Chinese Lifeworld*. Honolulu: University of Hawai'i Press.
https://doi.org/10.21313/hawaii/9780824835323.001.0001

Chan, K. Y. 1989. 'Joss Stick Manufacturing: A Study of a Traditional Industry in Hong Kong', *Journal of the Royal Asiatic Society Hong Kong Branch* 29: 94–120.

Chau, A. Y. 2006. *Miraculous Response – Doing Popular Religion in Contemporary China*. Stanford: Stanford University Press.

Chau, A. Y. 2008. 'The Sensorial Production of the Social', *Ethnos* 73.4: 485–504. https://doi.org/10.1080/00141840802563931

Chen, Y. 2013. 'The Perfume Culture of China and Taiwan: A Personal Report', *Journal of the Royal Asiatic Society* Series 3, 23.1, 127–130. https://doi.org/10.1017/S1356186313000059

Chiang, K.-C., and Liao, C.-M. 2006. 'Heavy Incense Burning in Temples Promotes Exposure Risk from Airborne PMs and Carcinogenic PAHs', *Science of the Total Environment* 372: 64–75. https://doi.org/10.1016/j.scitotenv.2006.08.012

Classen, C., Howes, D., and Synnott, A. 1994. *Aroma: The Cultural History of Smell*. New York: Routledge.

Clements, A. 2014. 'Divine Scents and Presence' in M. Bradley (ed.), *Smell and the Ancient Senses*. Florence: Taylor and Francis. pp. 46–59.

Corbett, J. M. 2006. 'Scents of Identity: Organisation Studies and the Cultural Conundrum of the Nose', *Culture and Organization* 12.3: 221–232. https://doi.org/10.1080/14759550600871469

Dannaway, F. R. 2010. 'Strange Fires, Weird Smokes and Psychoactive Combustibles: Entheogens and Incense in Ancient Traditions', *Journal of Psychoactive Drugs* 42.4: 485–497. https://doi.org/10.1080/02791072.2010.10400711

Doolittle, J. 1870. 'Ethnology: Sketches of Life in China. Incense Manufacture, Chinese Servants', *The Phrenological Journal of Science and Health (1870–1911)* 50.4: 236.

Feng, H. 2011. 'Politeness (Keqi): The Fragrance of Chinese Communication', *China Media Research* 7.4: 53–60.

Harvey, G. 2012. 'History of Animism (Part 3/8)'. Interview with Daniel Foor of Voices of the Earth. https://www.youtube.com/watch?v=ZnJVwyjRBng (last accessed 25 January 2017).

Harvey, G. 2013. *Food, Sex and Strangers: Understanding Religion as Everyday Life*. New York: Routledge.

Hashim, Y. Z., Kerr, P. G., Abbas, P., and Mohd Salleh, H. 2016. '*Aquilaria* spp. (Agarwood) as Source of Health Beneficial Compounds: A Review of Traditional Use, Phytochemistry and Pharmacology', *Journal of Ethnopharmacology* 189: 331–360. https://doi.org/10.1016/j.jep.2016.06.055

Henshaw, V. 2013. *Urban Smellscapes: Understanding and Designing City Smell Environments*. Florence: Taylor and Francis.

Henshaw, V. 2014. 'Welcome to the Smellscape', *New Scientist*, June 7: 28–29.

Jackson, D. D. 2011. 'Scents of Place: The Dysplacement of a First Nations Community in Canada', *American Anthropologist* 113.4: 606–618. https://doi.org/10.1111/j.1548-1433.2011.01373.x

Jochim, C. 1990. 'Flowers, Fruit, and Incense Only: Elite versus Popular in Taiwan's Religion of the Yellow Emperor', *Modern China* 16.1: 3–38. https://doi.org/10.1177/009770049001600101

Jung, D. 2013. 'The Cultural Biography of Agarwood – Perfumery in Eastern Asia and the Asian Neighborhood', *Journal of Royal Asiatic Society* Series 3, 23.1: 103–125. https://doi.org/10.1017/S1356186313000047

Lap, A. T., Yu, I. T., Qiu, H., Au, J. S., and Wang, X.-R. 2011. 'A Case-Referent Study of Lung Cancer and Incense Smoke, Smoking, and Residential Radon in Chinese Men', *Environmental Health Perspectives* 119.11: 1641–1646.
https://doi.org/10.1289/ehp.1002790

Lin, T.-C., Krishnaswamy, G., and Chi, D. S. 2008. 'Incense Smoke: Clinical, Structural, and Molecular Effects on Airway Disease', *Clinical and Molecular Allergy* 6: 3.
https://doi.org/10.1186/1476-7961-6-3

Low, K. E. Y. 2009. *Scent and Scent-sibilities: Smell and Everyday Life Experiences (1)*. Newcastle-Upon-Tyne: Cambridge Scholars Publishing.

McHugh, J. 2011. 'Seeing Scents: Methodological Reflection on the Intersensory Perception of Aromatics in South Asian Religions', *History of Religions* 51.2: 156–177. https://doi.org/10.1086/660930

Milburn, O. 2016. 'Aromas, Scents, and Spices: Olfactory Culture in China before the Arrival of Buddhism', *Journal of the American Oriental Society* 136.3: 441–464.
https://doi.org/10.7817/jameroriesoci.136.3.0441

Miyoshi, T., Ito, M., Kitayama, T., Isomori, S., and Yamashita, F. 2013. 'Sedative Effects of Inhaled Benzylacetone and Structural Features Contributing to Its Activity', *Biological and Pharmaceutical Bulletin* 36.9: 1474–1481.
https://doi.org/10.1248/bpb.b13-00250

Moeran, B. 2009. 'Making Scents of Smell: Manufacturing and Consuming Incense in Japan', *Human Organization* 68.4: 439–450.

Mohagheghzadeh, A., Faridi, P., Shams-Ardakani, M., and Ghasemi, Y. 2006. 'Medicinal Smokes: Review', *Journal of Ethnopharmacology* 108: 161–184.
https://doi.org/10.1016/j.jep.2006.09.005

Navasumrit, P., Arayasiri, M., Hiang, O.M., Leechawengwongs, M., Promvijit, J., Choonvisase, S., Chantchaemsai, S., Nakngam, N., Mahidol, M., and Ruchirawat, M. 2008. 'Potential Health Effects of Exposure to Carcinogenic Compounds in Incense Smoke in Temple Workers', *Chemico-Biological Interactions* 173.1: 19–31.
https://doi.org/10.1016/j.cbi.2008.02.004

Peace Rhind, J. 2013. *Fragrance and Wellbeing: Plant Aromatics and Their Influence on the Psyche*. London: Jessica Kingsley.

Rahim, H. 2005. 'Incense' in *Encyclopedia of Religion* (2nd edition). pp. 4418–4420.

Rasmussen, S. 1999. 'Making Better "Scents" in Anthropology: Aroma in Tuareg Sociocultural Systems and the Shaping of Ethnography', *Anthropological Quarterly* 72.2: 55–73. https://doi.org/10.2307/3317964

Reinarz, J. 2014. *Past Scents: Historical Perspectives on Smell*. Champaign: University of Illinois Press.

Rodaway, P. 2002. *Sensuous Geographies: Body, Sense, and Place*. London: Taylor and Francis.

Seow, W. J., and Lan, Q. 2016. 'Domestic Incense Use and Lung Cancer in Asia: A Review', *Reviews in Environmental Health* 31.1: 155–158.
https://doi.org/10.1515/reveh-2015-0060

Siripanich, S., Siriwong, W., Keawrueang, P., Borjan, M., and Robson, M. 2014. 'Incense and Joss Sticks Making in Small Household Factories, Thailand', *International Journal of Occupational and Environmental Medicine* 5.3: 137–145.

Staub, P. O., Geck, M. S., and Weckerle, C. S. 2011. 'Incense and Ritual Plant Use in Southwest China: A Case Study among the Bai in Shaxi', *Journal of Ethnobiology and Ethnomedicine* 7.43: 1–16. https://doi.org/10.1186/1746-4269-7-43

ter Haar, B. J. 1999. 'Teaching with Incense', *Studies of Central and East Asian Religions* 11: 1–14.

Yao, X., and Zhao, Y. 2010. *Chinese Religion: A Contextual Approach*. New York: Continuum.

Zavidovskaya, E. A. 2012. 'Deserving Divine Protection: Religious Life in Contemporary Rural Shanxi and Shaanxi Provinces', *St. Petersburg Annual of Asian and African Studies* 1: 179–197.

Shawn Arthur is an Assistant Professor in the Department of for the Study of Religions at Wake Forest University, Winston-Salem, NC, USA. His first book, *Early Daoist Dietary Practices: Examining Ways to Health and Longevity* (Lexington Books, 2013), focuses on a fifth-century Daoist text that contains recipes for achieving immortality. His current research focuses on contemporary popular religion in China and how lay practices and ideas can contribute to our understandings of 'religion' from non-official perspectives.

Section Two

TASTE

Chapter 3

The Taste of Religion in the Roman World

ZENA KAMASH[1]

It is late summer and the days are beginning to shorten: time for our yearly festival to Mercury. I walk up the hill past the meadows filled with young goats nibbling on sweet hay, soon to be dinner for Mercury. As I make my way to our feasting space, I'm salivating at the thought of the lamb ribs sprinkled with celery seeds; I just hope that the mulberries are riper this year as I can still taste their too-sour burst from last year. I look forward to this every year – a nice change from our usual beef and pork.

The cross-cultural close relationship between food and religion has long been noted (see Norman 2012 for an overview). In this chapter, I will explore the complexities of this relationship in the Roman world. I will start with a discussion of how to define taste. I will then briefly explain for those who are not specialists in archaeology and ancient history what kinds of evidence we have available to us and how we might use them to best effect.

---

1 I would first like to thank the editors, Jess and Graham, for inviting me to be part of this project and for their patience in the editorial process. In addition, the other contributors to the book helped in the shaping of the ideas expressed here, especially during productive discussions at our writing workshop in summer 2016. Tony King generously allowed me to use his tripole graphs as illustrations in my article, for which I am grateful. Priscilla Lange kindly shared her deep knowledge of animal bone and helped with several references. Finally, thanks must go to the gently frothy, slightly bitter flat whites and the comforting, melting sweetness of chocolate whose tastes largely fuelled the writing of this chapter.

Mainstream Roman religious practice relating to sacrifice and feasting has been well studied (see for example Beard et al. 1998; Scheid 2007; on the sensory experience of sacrifice see Weddle 2013 and 2017), so I will provide only a short overview of this below. The main analyses presented in this chapter draw on examples from the wider Roman Empire, principally the northwestern provinces (modern-day Britain and western Europe) and the Middle East. I will highlight some of the specific tastes of Roman religion, drawing out both how these differed from everyday life, and also how they differed from god to god and from god to human.

One of the key threads that runs through all the discussions in this chapter is that taste is nuanced and slippery. Taste does not play a simple game and therefore any exploration of it must allow for these complexities. This brings us, then, to an attempt to answer the question: what is taste?

WHAT IS TASTE?

The answer to this question is not as simple as it appears: it spans biology, chemistry and, crucially, culture. For these reasons, Korsmeyer (2007a: 1) characterizes it as being ambivalent and paradoxical, its status having been debated over many centuries. Chemically and biologically, taste traditionally comprises four categories: sweet, salty, bitter and sour. Even these categories, though, are open to challenge, with other contenders including metallic, alkaline and umami (Bartoshuk and Duffy 2007: 25). The classic tongue-map showing regions of the tongue associated with these sensations has now been proven false (ibid.: 27); instead all taste buds are equally able to taste these sensations (whatever we choose to put on our list). Moving from taste, strictly defined, to flavour, it is not only the taste buds that produce the sensation, but also the nose, via retronasal olfaction, whereby odorants are sensed as food is chewed and swallowed (ibid.).

Herein lies one of the paradoxes of taste: that it is not a single sense, but an intersense that must exist alongside smell and touch (and, arguably, vision as well, hence the effort made by modern chefs in food presentation). Sutton (2007: 312) has discussed this intersensoriality in terms of synaesthesia, by which he means 'the way that different senses elaborate on each other, rather than being considered separate domains of experience'. One of the best and oft-quoted examples of this intersensoriality comes from Proust's madeleine, where taste is intimately intertwined with smell, touch and, to a lesser extent, vision to create the hard-to-catch memory of Sunday mornings in Combray.

In addition, our tastes, our likes and our dislikes, are deeply affected by our upbringing and our cultural background. The tastes we like and dislike are a selection of 'that-which-can-conceivably-be-eaten' in a given culture (in the UK: cattle, sheep and pig are acceptable, but not dog or cat) made from 'all-that-is-possible-to-eat' (which includes cattle, sheep, pig, dog and cat) (James 2007: 374). This means that encounters with new foods can lead to fear and hesitation (Rozin and Rozin 2007: 38). Yet, in another paradox, cultural tastes are not fixed and can change over time. This was illustrated in the 2015 exhibition on Roman food which I curated at the Corinium Museum, Cirencester, where visitors were invited to share their food memories with us (https://notjustdormice.wordpress.com/food-memories/). Several memories mentioned trying out new foods, particularly curry or spicy foods. Here the initial attempt was often associated with a negative memory: 'My food memory relates to the first time I recall eating curry. My sister tried lime pickle and was so shocked by the heat that she threw flowers from the table and drank the cool water inside' (no. 125); 'My first chilli [sic] I was about 5–6 and spat it out.' (no. 269). Yet, no. 321 was brave enough to try again: 'Always try food you once dismissed as a child. I Hated [sic] curry with a vengancy [sic]. Curries are now one of my favourite things. I only started eating them at 37.'

This overview of taste leaves us, then, with a sense that is both particular to an individual, but also culturally constructed; a sense in its own right, but also intersensorial; culturally bounded, but also flexible and able to change over time.

EXCAVATING TASTE: FROM FOOD TO FLAVOUR

Since the post-processual turn in archaeology in the 1990s, the idea of archaeologies of the senses has become more widely accepted and mainstream (see e.g. Day 2013; Hamilakis 2013; Betts 2017). Some senses appear easier to reconstruct, for example, vision. Others, like taste, pose a few more challenges. In the introduction to her book on taste, Korsmeyer (2007a: 4) suggests that the 'tastes of history are elusive' and that any research 'must be supplemented by the imagination'. While I can understand such caution (and would be tempted to argue that, if we are honest, most attempts to understand the past require a healthy dose of imagination), I am inclined to be more hopeful about the possibility of understanding taste in the Roman period. Firstly, let us look at what evidence we have and what we might do with it.

There is some literary evidence at our disposal; for example, the fictional account of a lavish banquet thrown by the freedman Trimalchio (Petronius *Satyricon*[2]) and the so-called 'cookbook' attributed to Apicius, which is more likely a collection drawn from many sources (see Grocock and Grainger 2006). The latter is excellent for ingredients, but neither of the two is wholly reliable and both are often misused to focus on the weird (like roasted flamingo in Apicius 6.2.10) rather than the normal fruits, vegetables and pulses. In addition to these, writers like Pliny, Varro, Columella and Cato[3] give us insights into food production and, in some cases, clues as to the effects of those products. For example, Pliny (*Natural History* 14.8.6) tells us that wine from Pompeii can give you a headache that lasts until the sixth hour of the following day. I suspect many of us know how that sort of wine tastes.

More plentiful, though not without challenge, are the archaeological data on taste and religion. These data principally come from animal bones, plant remains and material culture associated with eating and drinking, such as ceramic tablewares, as well as stomach contents, coprolites and, more recently, isotopes. We can broadly split these into direct and indirect forms of evidence, where the latter (animal bones, plant remains and material culture) require more proof and inference to link them to food. Furthermore, these data provide insights into diet or meals, but rarely both. Meals, from stomach contents and coprolites, tend to be rare and found under very specific conditions, such as peat bogs. This raises questions: a bog body, for example, might have its stomach contents preserved, but how did it get there and how does this affect what was in its stomach? In the case of the bog body, Lindow Man, he seems to have been brutally killed, in fact overkilled, so he did not meet a natural death. His final meal included mistletoe (Brothwell 1986: 95-96), which is poisonous, so unlikely to be consumed as part of a normal diet. His violent death and his unusual stomach contents suggest that he might have been killed as part of a ritual.

The indirect evidence tends to provide evidence for diet rather than meals. There are three issues, not all negative, to bear in mind. First, while the evidence tends to preserve well in the archaeological record, good

---

2 Petronius *Satyricon* – Ruden, S. (ed.) 2000, Indianapolis: Hackett.
3 Pliny *Natural History* – Rackham, H. (ed.) 1969, London: Heinemann; Varro *On Agriculture* – Hooper, W. D., and Ash, H. B. (eds) 1934, London: Heinemann; Columella *On Agriculture* – Forster, E. S., and Heffner, E. H. (eds) 1955, London: Heinemann; Cato *On Agriculture* – Hooper, W. D., and Ash, H. B. (eds) 1934, London: Heinemann.

practice over the processing, recording and analysis of plant and animal remains has not always been undertaken. This has the effect of rendering many early excavations less helpful than they might have been (King 2005: 329). On the positive side, the subdisciplines of zooarchaeology and environmental archaeology have gained traction, so the quality and quantity of the data have risen and modern excavations now report on these assemblages routinely.

Second, we need to move an inferential step further with this evidence from food to flavour. This requires us to think beyond the material as it preserves to its implications. Plant remains are easiest here: we can see flavours through spices like pepper, for example. Open, ceramic platters lend themselves to dry roasts or joints of meat, whereas jars are better for stews. Similarly, young kill-off ages of sheep point to grilling or roasting as these methods are best suited to meat of this age, whereas later kill-off ages might point to slower cooking in a stew. These differing methods of cooking will have an inevitable effect on flavour profiles, and impact on the synaesthetic effect of the foods: slippery stew versus dry and firm roast.

Finally, using indirect evidence for diets rather than direct evidence for meals tends to mean that we are dealing with collectives rather than individuals (which is commonly the case in archaeology). The plus side of this is that we are well placed to track change (or lack of change) over time. This means that we are, primarily, looking at one facet of taste – cultural taste. I will, first, provide a brief overview of food and religion in the Roman world, before looking at some of the specificities of tastes in Roman religion.

FOOD AND ROMAN RELIGION: AN OVERVIEW

Roman religion and food were linked in two, related ways: food for the gods via sacrifices and food for the worshippers via feasting and dining, usually after the sacrifice. Sacrifices could be of incense, liquid libations, animals and of vegetal matter (Scheid 2007: 263). Vegetal offerings could be made of spelt (*far*), barley porridge (*polenta*), leavened bread, figs, cheeses, spelt porridge (*alica*), sesame and oil (ibid.: 265). A popular combination of animals for sacrifice was the *suovetaurilia*: pig, sheep and bull (Beard et al. 1998 [vol. 1]: 113, 327). Not all gods shared these tastes, though, as we will see below, and the particulars of any sacrifice were influenced by the ritual context with a wide range of different procedures (Scheid 2007: 263,

267). In preparation for their sacrifice, the back of the animal victim would be scattered with *mola salsa* (salted flour – salt is discussed further below), wine poured on their forehead and then a knife passed over their back (ibid.: 266; also see Weddle 2017: 347–357 for a discussion of touch in these actions). The divinity's portion would then be cooked in a pot (cattle) or roasted on a spit (sheep and pigs) (Scheid 2007: 266). When ready to be served to the god, the portion was sprinkled with more *mola salsa* and wine. It could then be burned on the altar or plunged into water for aquatic deities or served on a table in a *lectisternium* ritual. The *lectisternium*, which is first known in the Roman world from 399 BCE, comprised statues of gods or their attributes placed on dining couches (*puluinaria*) to consume offerings that had been laid out on a table (Beard et al. 1998 [vol. 2]: 130; Scheid 2007: 266; Livy *History*[4] V.13.5–8). These couches and tables became popular as permanent features in temples from the first century CE onwards (Scheid 2007: 267). Some of the banquets could be quite elaborate; for example, those of the *Fratres Arvales*, a college of priests to the Goddess Ceres, were composed of two courses: a meat course, followed by a course of sweetened wine and cake (ibid.; Weddle 2017: 374–378). After the divinity had eaten, those performing the sacrifice would usually then eat. It seems that mortals and immortals deliberately did not eat the same meals, in order to maintain their division and hierarchy (Beard et al. 1998 [vol. 1]: 36–37; Veyne 2000: 6). Evidence for the tastes of the worshippers will be discussed in more detail below, with specific attention to where these diverge from the tastes of the gods, as well as from mundane tastes.

THE DIFFERENT TASTES OF ROMAN RELIGION

There is evidence to suggest that Roman religion may have tasted differently to other aspects of Roman daily life. This is particularly clear in evidence from Roman Britain where animal bone evidence suggests that the food consumed at Romano-British religious sites was different to those consumed in other contexts (King 2005: 331–332). The tripole graph in Figure 3.1 shows the consumption of different kinds of animals across a broad range of settlement types in Roman Britain. From this graph we can see that cattle (domestic ox) and pig were consumed in higher quantities in urban and military sites, including legionary sites. In rural settlements, there was a greater dependency on sheep/goat and so higher continuity

---

4 Livy *History* – Foster, O.B. (ed.) 1919, London: Heinemann.

The Taste of Religion in the Roman World   69

with pre-Roman food profiles (note that 'sheep/goat' is a commonly-used term by archaeologists as it is often difficult to identify one species from the other; this term will be used throughout, unless it has been possible to distinguish the species). The temple sites, which are plotted in Figure 3.2, broadly show a similar pattern, but with a cluster in the lower right-hand corner of the graph that is not present on other site types. This cluster of temples has high sheep/goat numbers and low numbers of cattle and pig. In this case the emphasis on sheep/goat is higher than on rural sites and suggests that certain temple sites had very particular tastes. This gives us a tantalizing glimpse into the distinctiveness of religious taste in the Roman world. In what follows, I will explore what some of these distinctive religious tastes might have been, including some of the animal bone evidence

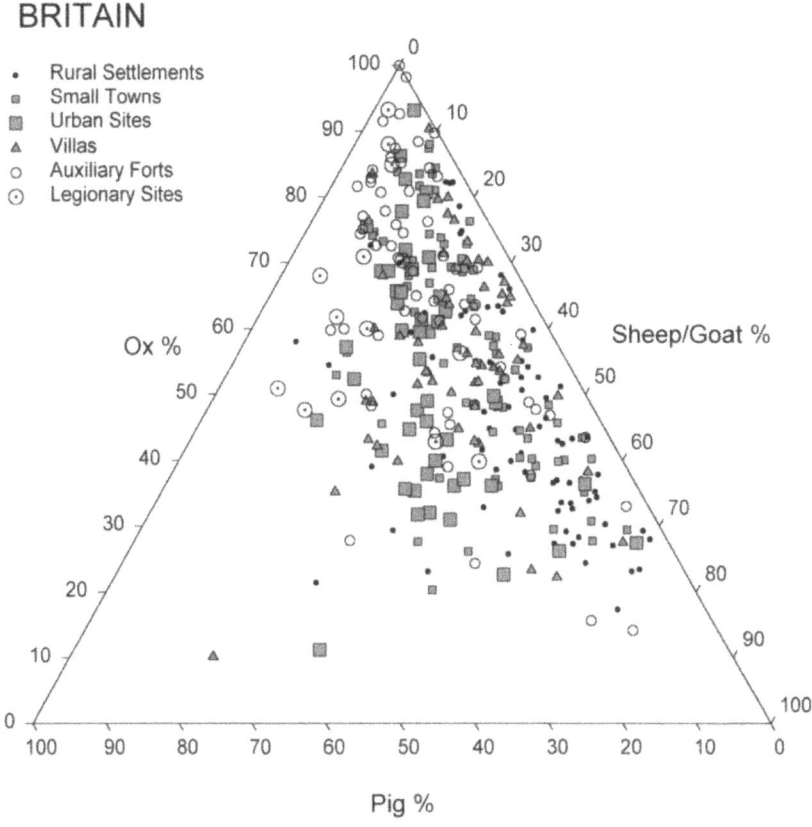

Figure 3.1 Tripole graph showing percentages of domestic ox, sheep/goat and pig for all site types in Roman Britain. From King 2005: fig. 2.

TEMPLES IN ROMAN BRITAIN

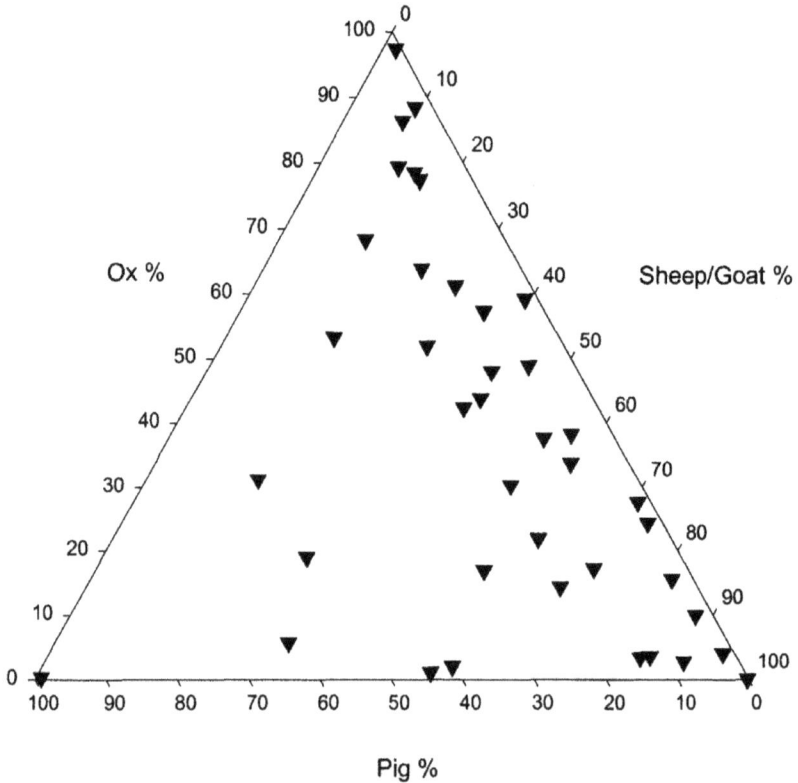

Figure 3.2 Tripole graph showing percentages of domestic ox, sheep/goat and pig for Romano-British temple sites. From King 2005: fig. 3.

referred to here. Some of these, such as the honeyed cakes, seem to be fairly widespread in Roman religion, whereas others seem to denote the tastes of specific gods and rituals. In addition, while we can identify some of the quartet of tastes (sweet, salty, bitter and sour), other tastes seem to fall outside of those strict categories, such as goat-y at Uley or chicken-y in *mithraea* (temples to Mithras).

Sweet, bitter and floral

Some recipes from the literary sources are specific to Roman religion, in particular recipes for two cakes: *libum* and *placenta* (the latter term translates as 'flat cake' and does not have a connection to birth in the Roman world). The recipes for these cakes are found in Cato *De Agricultura* 75–76. The recipe for *libum* is brief and comprises cheese and flour. The recipe for *placenta* is more detailed and provides more evidence for the taste of these cakes. Most notably these cakes are sweetened *cum melle*, 'with honey' included in the cheese and flour mixture and drizzled on after baking. The addition of the honey seems to be key to the flavour, making it distinctively religious. In Horace *Epistles*[5] 1.10.10–11 we hear of a priest's runaway slave who rejects his former food and longs for plain bread, rather than *mellitis placentis* ('honeyed cakes').

The taste of these cakes would have come not only from the deep sweetness of the honey as an ingredient, but also from the method of cooking. Cato specifies that the *placenta* should be baked on a bed of oiled bay leaves (*folia laurea uncta supponito*). The same specification for this particular leaf is also found throughout Apicius (Grocock and Grainger 2006: 347). The bed of leaves would have prevented the cakes from burning on the bottom while baking, but would also have imparted the bitter taste and floral scent of bay to the cakes. The inclusion of a bitter taste is interesting as in other contexts it is associated with cursing. For example, in the Old Testament 'bitter waters' are prescribed as a curse for an adulterous woman (Numbers 5:11–31).

Salty

Salt seems to have held a special place in ritual and religious ceremonies, as we have already seen above with *mola salsa*. Studies on the significance of salt have suggested that its symbolic importance derives from its ability to prevent decay. It is therefore hated by devils and demons, hence the superstition of throwing salt over your left shoulder (Jones 1923: 116; Visser 1986: 77). In addition, due to its association with purity, it is often linked with powerful substances like iron or blood, especially in oath-taking rituals (ibid.: 75, 77). In the Old Testament references are made to its use in offerings: for example, worshippers are instructed to season their grain offerings with salt (Leviticus 2.13); similarly, we are told that when young bulls without blemish are made as a burnt offering, priests shall throw salt on them (Ezekiel 43.24).

---

5 Horace *Epistles* – Dilke, O.A.W. (ed.) 1954, London: Methuen.

In the Roman period there are glimpses of salt, specifically saltwater, playing an important role in rituals. In his second century CE treatise on Dea Syria ('the Syrian goddess'), Lucian makes reference to water-pouring rituals (*De Dea Syria* [*DDS*] 13, 48, see Lightfoot 2003). In both cases, he specifies that the water is brought from the sea; in *DDS* 48 he states that the ritual is part of a festival by the sea. Lightfoot (2003: 350), who rightly notes that Lucian is not always a reliable source, queries this insistence on seawater as the main cult site for Dea Syria at Hierapolis in Syria is a long journey from the Mediterranean sea (the closest source of seawater). As I have argued elsewhere, however, the story is not implausible given the inland trade in Mediterranean fish products and the general ritual significance of salt and so, by extension, saltwater (Kamash 2010: 173). In addition, we also know of another case of seawater used in rituals near Hierapolis from the *Apology* of Pseudo-Meliton (Lightfoot 2007: 84, 99–105). In this account, magicians use seawater to slay the unclean demon living in a well, which again is similar to the other known uses of salt in ritual outlined above.

These stories all suggest that salt has played a key role in ritual and religion, including during the Roman period. While salt in some of these cases may not have been consumed by worshippers, it may be seen as part of the taste of the gods. As such, we might postulate a formula where salty equals godly, while unsalty equals ungodly.

THE TASTES OF MERCURY AT ULEY

One of the sites that sits in the corner of the tripole graph in Figure 3.2 is Uley in Gloucestershire, UK. Uley is a large temple complex that has a long history, spanning eight centuries, developing from a small shrine in the early first century CE to a large complex with multiple buildings in the second century to early fourth century CE before converting from paganism to Christianity in the fifth to sixth century CE (Woodward and Leach 1993: 10–11). The temple was dedicated to the god Mercury, whose attributes include a goat and a cockerel. The site was well excavated and produced a large animal bone assemblage (a total of 232,322 fragments), studied by Bruce Levitan (1993).

The most striking facet of the animal bone assemblage is its extremely high proportion of sheep/goat, up to 90 percent in some phases, as well as a higher than usual proportion of domestic fowl (Levitan 1993: 257–258). Furthermore, of the sheep/goat bones, the majority could be confidently identified at species level as goat, which makes the assemblage highly unusual (ibid.: 258). In what follows, I will focus on the animal bone assemblage from four buildings: Structures IV and X from Phase 4 (second to third century CE) and Structures I and IX from Phase 5 (mid-fourth century CE). In each phase there are distinctive differences in the animal bone assemblages between the building in each pair that suggest that one building was used for food for Mercury and one was used for food consumed by the worshippers. This provides us with an excellent opportunity to explore the differing tastes of these two sets of consumers at Uley. Data for the animal bones discussed below are drawn from Levitan (1993: 266–288).

In all four buildings the majority of the animal bone assemblage comprises sheep/goat with a negligible contribution from cattle and pig, and a small, but significant, amount of domestic fowl (i.e. a higher proportion than might be expected from comparative assemblages). Within this broad pattern, which already marks Uley out as unusual, there are nuanced differences across the buildings in terms of kill-off ages, sexing and butchery.

In the Phase 4 building, Structure IV, goats predominated. Most parts of the anatomy were present and evidence for butchery was rare: 1 percent in Phase 4a and 0.6 percent in Phase 4b. This suggests strongly that these goats were not consumed by worshippers, though Cool (2006: 211) raises the possibility of spit-roasting. The likelihood that these goats were intended for Mercury is highlighted by a preference for male animals and a young kill-off age, potentially indicating a need for unblemished animals for sacrifice. The specificity of the kill-off ages at 6, 18 and 30 months suggests that the animals were killed once a year, probably in August or September. The animal bone assemblage as a whole corroborates this idea of a major, annual summer festival for Mercury at Uley.

Structure X shows some key differences to the contemporary Structure IV. First, sheep were more common in Structure X with a sheep:goat ratio of 6:5 (in contrast to 1:3 in Structure IV). This suggests that while goats were exclusively food for Mercury, the worshippers' food was more sheep-y than goat-y. Secondly, there was a greater frequency of butchery marks on the Structure X bones – 6–10 percent – pointing to the division of the carcass into portions for eating. While the animals showed the same annual kill-off patterns, the age range of the animals was slightly broader at up to three years, suggesting less need for young, unblemished animals. Both structures also had evidence for domestic fowl, but differences between the buildings in this part of the assemblage are harder to find.

In Phase 5, in the mid-fourth century CE, Structure IV was joined by Structure I, which in many ways continued the roles of Structure IV, but with sheep/goat making up an even higher proportion of the animal bone assemblage and with over 70 percent of the assemblage being goat for Mercury. As in Structure IV almost all parts of the goat were represented, but very little of it – less than 1 percent – was butchered. Where butchery was present, it was predominantly on horncores and so unlikely to be associated with food consumption (Priscilla Lange pers. comm.). Again males predominated in both sheep and goat. In contrast to Structure IV, domestic fowl show a decrease over time from 4.5 percent at the beginning of Phase 5 to 1.6 percent later on.

Structure IX replaced Structure X in Phase 5 and, similarly, echoed the roles of its predecessor. Sheep/goat still make up the majority of the assemblage, rising from 80 percent to 90 percent, but in stark contrast to Structure I, sheep, rather than goat, dominate the assemblage at 70 percent. There is also a larger amount of butchery evidence on 2–4 percent of the bones. In this case, the butchery marks were concentrated on ribs and then on upper limbs and girdles. This seems to echo the sheep-y tastes for worshippers in Phase 4. Another difference to Structure I is that domestic fowl were present in larger numbers, though also decreasing over time from 8.9 percent to 5.9 percent. This raises the interesting possibility that Mercury had a taste preference for one of his cult animals over the other; while goat was almost exclusively for him, domestic fowl could be shared with his worshippers. In terms of body parts of domestic fowl, wings were most common, followed by legs, head and body. This evidence evokes images of worshippers nibbling stickily on a rack of ribs as well as chicken wings and thighs during their late summer feast.

Structure IX also gives us tantalizing glimpses of some of the flavours accompanying this feast of ribs and wings. This evidence comes from a latrine pit, which had good conditions for the survival of plant remains (Girling and Straker 1993: 252). Locally available plants included apples, blackberries and elder. Mulberries were also found; although not native to the UK, as the fruit need to be eaten fully ripe some trees must have been grown here (Cool 2006: 122). Even when ripe, mulberries are a very sour fruit (giving us the final part of the taste quartet!). Celery seeds, which were probably traded, were also found, which were a common flavouring in sauces, for example for crane, duck or chicken (Apicius 6.2.2), for boiled partridge, francolin and turtle-dove (Apicius 6.2.7) and for 'all kinds of boiled and roast game' (Apicius 8.4.2: *ius in uenationibus omnibus elixis et assis*). We even get to see the tastes of the animals being consumed by Mercury and his worshippers through the plant-remains evidence for sweet hay cut from managed grassland, suggesting that the animals were brought alive to the temple and kept there briefly before sacrifice.

The Taste of Religion in the Roman World 75

In summary, then, we get a vivid taste picture from Uley of distinctive taste profiles for the god Mercury, who seems to have enjoyed a diet of young male goat. In contrast, the feasts of his worshippers comprised a broader, but still not mundane, range of tastes of sheep, goat and chicken, flavoured with celery seeds and accompanied by sour and fruity flavours of apple, blackberries and mulberries.

THE TASTES OF MITHRAS

Mithraism was a Roman mystery cult, whose central myth related to Mithras killing a bull and the victory of light over dark. While not a mainstream part of Roman religion, *mithraea* (temples to Mithras) are known from across the Roman world (for a useful bibliography on Mithraism see Martens and De Boe 2004). These *mithraea* took a distinctly different form to traditional Roman temples; they were supposed to resemble caves and had a pair of benches running parallel either side of a central aisle towards an altar at the far end.

In the past couple of decades, several high-quality excavations have taken place at *mithraea*, in which large animal bone assemblages have been excavated. One of the most significant of these is the third century CE *mithraeum* at Tienen, Belgium (Martens et al. 2004). This site is particularly noteworthy because it includes a series of pits, which were filled by the debris of a single large feasting event in the second half of the third century CE (Lentacker et al. 2004: 57). The ceramic and animal bone assemblages point to c. 100 people having participated at this feast (Martens et al. 2004: 43). The numbers of plates (85), colour-coated beakers (79) and jars (80) suggests that each participant had their own set of crockery for the feast (ceramic numbers from ibid.: 32): a plate, a jar and a beaker. In addition, there were three larger beakers for mixing, which point to a communal element to the feast. The plant remains from the pits were limited, and may not all derive from the feast, but what is present points to the consumption of cereals (spelt, with some barley and possibly emmer), as well as lentils, hazelnuts and elder (ibid.: 49). Some carbonized fragments of a processed food (too small to be analysed in more depth) were also found, which might have been bread, but possibly also broth or porridge (ibid.). It is tempting to suppose these remains were of broth or porridge that was served in the jars as part of the feast.

As at Uley, the animal bone assemblage presents particularly good evidence for the tastes of Mithraism at Tienen. Firstly, the fishbone assemblage, especially the Spanish mackerel, points to the supplementing of the food at the feast with *salsamenta*: salted fish. *Salsamenta* was commonly produced and traded around the Mediterranean (Curtis 1991; Trakadas 2005: 69–72; Wilson 2006). In terms of flavour and sensory experience, the *salsamenta* would, of course, have been salty and fishy, but also chewy and slightly sweet; in modern cooking it is often used to bring out the flavour of the food it accompanies.

The most striking aspect of the Tienen animal bone assemblage is the extremely high number of domestic fowl (Table 3.1), which represents a minimum number of c. 265–285 individual chickens, with an MNI (Minimum Number of Individuals) of 83 subadults and 155 adults (Lentacker et al. 2004: 60). The burning on the chicken bones suggests that the adult birds were fried or roasted and subadults broiled on a spit.

The Tienen assemblage is also noteworthy for its very low number of cattle bones in comparison to the pig and sheep/goat bones. The sheep/goat and pig bones both seem to represent partially-preserved complete skeletons and both were killed off at very young ages (Lentacker et al. 2004: 65), again pointing to a preference for young animals for sacrifice and consumption on temple sites. The very young age of the pigs and sheep/goat suggest they were probably killed in June or July pointing to a feast in early summer (ibid.: 68). The MNI for the sheep/goat indicates 14 lambs, and for pigs 10 piglets (ibid.: 65). As with the chicken bones, the pig and sheep/

Table 3.1 Animal bone by fragment count by species from selected *mithraea*. Crypta Balbi in the seventh century was no longer a *mithraeum* and is included for comparative purposes. Data from – Tienen (large and small pits): Lentacker et al. 2004; Martigny and Orbe-Boscéaz: Olive 2004; Crpyta Balbi (both phases): Mazzorin 2004.

	Tienen - large pit	Tienen - small pits	Martigny	Orbe-Boscéaz	Crypta Balbi - final phase	Crytpa Balbi - seventh century
Domestic fowl	7,615	1,307	3,388	252	68	245
Pig	278	95	5,159	352	219	1,863
Sheep/goat	314	43	1,818	28	45	1,156
Cattle	77	78	515	121	16	240
Other	3,195	339	268	21	26	–
Unidentified	2,449	2,128	18,213	1,010	–	–
Total	13,928	3,990	29,361	1,784	374	3,504

goat bones displayed frequent burning, suggesting that they were spit-roasted (ibid.: 66–67).

In contrast, the cattle bones were from older animals and mostly represented by loose teeth and small fragments from large bones, which suggests that these were habitation refuse and probably not associated with the main feast (Lentacker et al. 2004: 65). This lack of cattle bones at the *mithraeum* becomes more significant when compared with the assemblage from the Zijdelingsestraat site in Tienen that provides a sample of general, everyday refuse. At this site, chicken, which were strongly represented at the *mithraeum*, are negligible, whereas cattle, which are so poorly represented in the *mithraeum* pits, are extremely high in the general refuse (ibid.: 69). This suggests that the foods consumed at the *mithraeum* are not similar to those the inhabitants of Tienen were eating on a daily basis and, furthermore, points strongly to a taboo over eating cattle at the *mithraeum*. As noted at the beginning of this section, bulls feature strongly in the iconography and mythology of the cult of Mithras, so it seems that this animal is too sacred to be eaten during a Mithraic feast. This temporary taboo on a particular foodstuff is similar, for example, to some Hindu festivals, which are declared as meatless days (Meyer-Rochow 2009).

If such a thing as a menu existed, then, for the Tienen *mithraeum*, it might have read something like: 'Mithras Fried Chicken; spit-roasted suckling pig and lamb served with *salsamenta*, elder and lentil broth. Hazelnuts are available for snacking. Under no circumstances may beef be eaten at this festival!'

There is evidence to suggest that these eating practices were widespread across *mithraea* and, therefore, that Mithraism could be said to have had a distinctive taste. As Table 3.1 shows, cattle are consistently low across the *mithraea* at Martigny (Switzerland), Orbe-Boscéaz (Switzerland) and Crypta Balbi (Rome). There is also a distinctive preference at these sites for chicken and pig with slightly lower consumption of sheep/goat. At Orbe-Boscéaz there is a seeming dislike for sheep/goat, which is at odds with the other sites and may reflect more personal preference as this is a rural *mithraeum* linked to a villa. In addition, at Crypta Balbi, the preference seems to be more for pig than chicken, though chicken was still being consumed in high numbers. This seems to be at odds with the general pattern for *mithraea* as there are hints from other sites for the importance of chicken, in particular, at Mithraic feasts, for example chicken was most common at the *mithraea* in London (Macready and Sidell 1998: 213), Carrawburgh in England (Richmond and Gillam 1951), Kugelstein in Austria (Adam et al. 1996), Aquincum in Hungary (Vörös 1991), Künzing in

Table 3.2 Kill-off ages in months of pig and sheep/goat by percentage of assemblage from Martigny *mithraeum* compared to the general area. Data from Olive 2004: table 2.

Martigny	Mithraeum		General area	
Age in months	Pig (n=184)	Sheep/goat (n=114)	Pig (n=20)	Sheep/goat (n=6)
3–6	35	25	9	15
6–12	39	18	15	20
12–24	15	23	36.5	20
24–36	6.5	16.5	27.5	30
36+	4.5	17.5	12	15

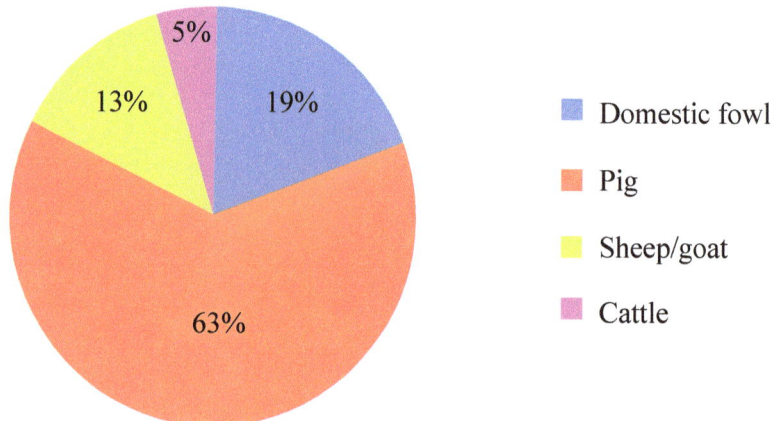

Figure 3.3 The final phase of the Crypta Balbi *mithraeum* animal assemblage by percentage of fragment count (not including the 'other' category as this was not provided by the report author for the seventh century CE). Data from Mazzorin 2004.

Germany (von den Driesch and Pöllath 2000) and made up 78 percent of the assemblage at the Septeuil *mithraeum* in France (Gaidon-Bunuel 2002). In addition, accounts from the *mithraeum* at Dura Europos in Syria mention the buying of fowl for ritual banquets (Richmond and Gillam 1951: 16 fn. 14–16). Lentacker et al. (2004: 72) suggest that this preference towards fowl may be related to their links with sunrise, which would fit with the emphasis on light versus dark seen in Mithraism.

Table 3.3 Kill-off ages in months of pig and sheep/goat by percentage of assemblage from Orbe-Boscéaz *mithraeum* compared to the Orbe-Boscéaz villa. Data from Olive 2004: table 2.

Orbe-Boscéaz	Mithraeum		Villa	
Age in months	Pig (n=20)	Sheep/goat (n=6)	Pig (n=39)	Sheep/goat (n=13)
3–6	25	50	15	15.3
6–12	60	33.5	4	54
12–24	15	16.5	41	15.3
24–36	–	–	29	15.3
36+	–	–	11	–

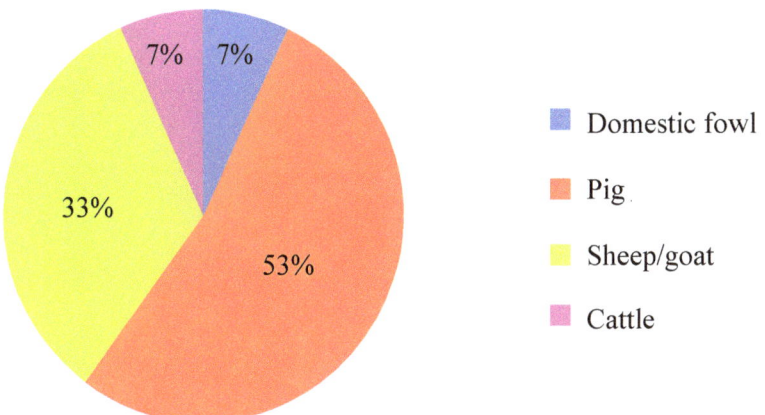

Figure 3.4 The animal bone assemblage from the seventh century CE occupation at Crypta Balbi by percentage of fragment count. Data from Mazzorin 2004.

Some of these sites also give us the chance to compare some of the elements of a Mithraic and a non-Mithraic assemblage. At Martigny and Orbe-Boscéaz, it is clear that younger animals were specifically chosen for consumption at the *mithraea* than was usual in the general consumption pattern (Tables 3.2 and 3.3). In both sites, pigs were killed off substantially earlier for the *mithraeum*: 74 percent vs 24 percent before 12 months at Martigny and 85 percent vs 19 percent before 12 months at

Orbe-Boscéaz. This suggests a preference for young pig, often suckling pig, as seen at Tienen above. The pattern is less strong for sheep/goat, but there seems to be a slight preference for lamb at both *mithraea*: 43 percent vs 35 percent before 12 months at Martigny and 83.5 percent vs 69.3 percent before 12 months at Orbe-Boscéaz. At Crypta Balbi, we can also see some distinct differences between the final phase of the *mithraeum* in the fifth century CE and the occupation on the site in the seventh century CE, with the preference for domestic fowl and pig dropping after the *mithraeum* goes out of use, and a slight rise in cattle consumption (Table 3.1 and Figures 3.3–3.4).

Overall, then, it appears that feasts at *mithraea* tasted distinctly different from meals eaten in daily life, with a seeming taboo on the consumption of beef that is not found on other sites. In addition, the very strong preference towards chicken seems not only to mark out Mithraism from daily life, but also from other religions in the Roman world, where chicken consumption was not unknown, but was rarely as high as in *mithraea* (Lentacker et al. 2004: 71). Furthermore, it seems that certain animals and tastes are included (chicken) or excluded (beef) in order to fit with the particularities of the Mithraic ideology, thus intimately linking taste with religious practice or doctrine in this context.

CONCLUSIONS

There are many more examples that could have been included here and many more sources to explore. This topic is clearly deserving of further study in order to better understand the nuances of taste and religion in the Roman world. In spite of this, I will attempt to answer the question that has been in my mind while writing this chapter: what did Roman religion taste like? In the simplest terms, it did not taste like daily life. What people ate at religious sites was not the same as what they ate at home or on the street. There appear to be numerous ways in which this difference could be expressed: through the eating of sweet, honeyed cakes; through the sprinkling of salt or pouring of saltwater; through the use of young, unblemished animals; through the deliberate selection of certain parts of an animal to eat; through the imposition of apparent taboos over the consumption of certain foodstuffs, particularly certain animals. Religious tastes, though, were not necessarily uniform, so the answer also has to be context-specific. Some tastes seem to have been specific to, and redolent of, certain religions: goat for Mercury; chicken for Mithras. By moving from food remains to flavour, by taking that additional inferential step, we can also start, even if in a 'tongue-in-cheek' way to think about particular menus that worshippers might have anticipated when visiting certain temples: ribs and wings at Uley; fried chicken at Mithras (and so, maybe Korsmeyer was right to say we need to use our imaginations). In some cases, as in Mithraism, these tastes were shared across space, so that one *mithraeum* tasted much like another *mithraeum*, strengthening bonds across the community of believers in Mithras. Religion, however, did not necessarily taste the same for gods and humans. This could be through the eating of different animals – goats for the gods and sheep for the humans at Uley. It seems that the only way to understand taste is to embrace its paradoxical nature and use this to illuminate the complexities of the relationship between taste and religion in the Roman world.

REFERENCES

Adam, A., Czeika, S., and Fladerer, F. A. 1996. 'Römerzeitliche Tierknochenfunde aus zwei Höhlen am Kugelstein bei Deutschfeistritz, Steiermark – Hinweise auf den Mithraskult?' *Mitteilungen Anthropologische Geselschaft Wien* 125–126: 279–289.

Bartoshuk, L. M., and Duffy, V. B. 2007. 'Chemical Senses: Taste and Smell' in Korsmeyer (2007: 25–33).

Beard, M., North, J., and Price, S. 1998. *Religions of Rome* (2 vols). Cambridge: Cambridge University Press.

Betts, E. (ed.) 2017. *Senses of the Empire: Multisensory Approaches to Roman Culture*, London: Routledge.

Brothwell, D. 1986. *The Bogman and the Archaeology of People*. London: British Museum Publications.

Cool, H. E. M. 2006. *Eating and Drinking in Roman Britain*. Cambridge: Cambridge University Press. https://doi.org/10.1017/CBO9780511489570

Curtis, R. I. 1991. *Garum and Salsamenta*. Leiden: Brill.

Day, J. (ed.) 2013. *Making Senses of the Past: Toward a Sensory Archaeology*. Carbondale: South Illinois University Press.

Gaidon-Bunuel, M-A. 2002. 'La cuisine du mithraeum de Septeuil' in S. Lepetz and W. van Andringa (eds), *Archéologie du sacrifice animal en Gaule romaine: Rituels et pratiques alimentaires, Volume des pré-actes*. Paris: Editions Monique Mergoil. pp. 70–83.

Girling, M., and Straker, V. 1993. 'Plant macrofossils, arthropods and charcoal' in Woodward and Leach (1993: 250–253).

Grocock, C., and Grainger, S. 2006. *Apicius: A Critical Edition with an Introduction and English Translation*. Totnes: Prospect Books.

Hamilakis, Y. (ed.) 2013. *Archaeology and the Senses: Human Experience, Memory and Affect*. Cambridge: Cambridge University Press. https://doi.org/10.1017/CBO9781139024655

James, A. 2007. 'Identity and the Global Stew' in Korsmeyer (2007: 372–384).
Jones, E. 1923. 'The Symbolic Significance of Salt in Folklore and Superstition' in E. Jones (ed.), *Essays in Applied Psycho-Analysis*. London: The International Psycho-Analytical Press. pp. 112–203.
Kamash, Z. 2010. *Archaeologies of Water in the Roman Near East*. New York: Gorgias Press.
King, A. 2005. 'Animal Remains from Temples in Roman Britain', *Britannia* 36: 329–369. https://doi.org/10.3815/000000005784016964
Korsmeyer, C. (ed.) 2007. *The Taste Culture Reader: Experiencing Food and Drink*. Oxford and New York: Berg.
Korsmeyer, C. 2007a. 'Introduction: Perspectives on Taste' in Korsmeyer (2007: 1–9).
Lentacker, A., Ervynck, A., and Van Neer, W. 2004. 'The Symbolic Meaning of the Cock: The Animal Remains from the *Mithraeum* at Tienen, Belgium' in Martens and De Boe (2004: 57–80).
Levitan, B. 1993. 'Vertebrate Remains' in Woodward and Leach (1993: 257–301).
Lightfoot, J. (ed.) 2003. *Lucian: on the Syrian Goddess*. Oxford: Oxford University Press.
Lightfoot, J. 2007. 'The Apology of Pseudo-Meliton,' *Studi Epigrafici e Linguistiti* 24: 59–110.
Macready, S., and Sidell, J. 1998. 'The Animal Bones' in J.D. Shepherd (ed.), *The Temple of Mithras*. London: English Heritage. pp. 208–15.
Martens, M., and De Boe, G. (eds). 2004. *Roman Mithraism: The Evidence of the Small Finds*. Brussels: Institute for the Archaeological Heritage of the Flemish Community (IAP).
Martens, M., with Cooremans, B., and Deforce, K. 2004. 'The *Mithraeum* at Tienen (Belgium): Small Finds and What They Can Tell Us' in Martens and De Boe (2004: 25–56).
Mazzorin, J. D. G. 2004. 'I resti animali del mitreo della Crypta Balbi: testimonianze di pratiche cultuali' in Martens and De Boe (2004: 179–82)
Meyer-Rochow, V. B. 2009. 'Food Taboos: Their Origins and Purposes', *Journal of Ethnobiology and Ethnomedicine* 5. https://doi.org/10.1186/1746-4269-5-18
Norman, C. E. 2012. 'Food and Religion' in J. M. Pilcher (ed.), *The Oxford Handbook of Food History*. Oxford: Oxford University Press. pp. 409–423.
Olive, C. 2004. 'La faune exhumée des *mithraea* de Martigny (Valais) et d'Orbe-Boscéaz (Vaud) en Suisse' in Martens and De Boe (2004: 147–156).
Richmond, I. A., and Gillam, J. P. 1951. 'The Temple of Mithras at Carrawburgh', *Archaeologia Aeliana* 29: 1–92.
Rozin, E., and Rozin, P. 2007. 'Culinary Themes and Variations' in Korsmeyer (2007: 34–41).
Scheid, J. 2007. 'Sacrifices for Gods and Ancestors' in Rüpke, J. (ed.), *A Companion to Roman Religion*. Malden MA: Blackwell. https://doi.org/10.1002/9780470690970.ch19
Sutton, D. E. 2007. 'Synesthesia, Memory and the Taste of Home' in Korsmeyer (2007: 304–316).
Trakadas, A. 2005. 'The Archaeological Evidence for Fish Processing in the Western Mediterranean' in T. Bekker-Nielsen (ed.), *Ancient Fishing and Fish Processing in the Black Sea Region*. Aarhus: Aarhus University Press. pp. 47–82.
Veyne, P. 2000. 'Inviter les dieux, sacrifier, banqueter: Quelques nuances de la religiosité romaine', *Annales Économie, Sociétés, Civilisations* 55: 3–42.
Visser, M. 1986 *Much Depends on Dinner*. New York: HarperCollins.

von den Driesch, A., and Pöllath, N. 2000. 'Tierknochen aus dem Mithrastempel von Künzing, Lkr. Deggendorf' in K. Schmotz (ed.), *Vorträge des 18. Niederbayerischen Archäologentages*. Rahden/Westfalen. pp. 145-162.

Vörös, I. 1991. 'Das Haus des Tribuni Laticlavii aus dem Legionslager vom 2-3 Jh in Aquincum. Das Tierknochenmaterial des Mithräums', *Budapest Régiségei* 28: 155.

Weddle, C. 2013. 'The Sensory Experience of Blood Sacrifice in the Roman Imperial Cult' in J. Day (ed.), *Making Senses of the Past: Toward a Sensory Archaeology*. Carbondale: Southern Illinois University Press. pp. 137-59.

Weddle, C. 2017. 'Blood, Fire and Feasting: The Role of Touch and Taste in Graeco-Roman Animal Sacrifice' in Betts (2017: 338-392).

Wilson, A. 2006. 'Fishy Business: Roman Exploitation of Marine Resources', *Journal of Roman Archaeology* 19: 525-537. https://doi.org/10.1017/S1047759400006760

Woodward, A., and Leach, P. 1993. *The Uley Shrines: Excavation of a Ritual Complex on West Hill, Uley, Gloucestershire: 1977-9*. London: English Heritage.

Zena Kamash is Lecturer in Roman Archaeology in the Department of Classics at Royal Holloway University of London, UK. She has wide-ranging interests that include food, religion and memory in the Roman world with a particular focus on Roman Britain and the Roman Middle East. She has curated an exhibition on food in the Roman world at Corinium Museum (Cirencester, UK).

CHAPTER 4

Candomblé's Eating Myths: Religion Stated in Food Language

PATRICIA RODRIGUES DE SOUZA

Food is my religion, the kitchen is my temple, and my sacred book contains recipes. This chapter is an invitation to Candomblé's kitchen, a place where devotion comes from its pans. In this African-Brazilian religion, humans and gods eat together. Gods have their favourite foods: beans, yams, sweet potato, okra, corn made in all forms, coconut, chillies, all sorts of meat ... all spiced with onion, and dried shrimps sautéed in rich colourful palm oil. Ceremonies are banquets with music, dancing and meaningful, elaborate foods. Everyone is invited, there's no need to be a practitioner, prosperity is to be shared.

From the very beginning of human history, religion and food have been related. Ancient cults had tutelary gods and goddesses of wheat, rice, grapes, cows and pigs – and they would all get fed and offered sacrifices. The Hebrew Bible contains a whole book (Leviticus) on dietary rules: what could or couldn't be eaten, when and in what manner, and with whom. As Graham Harvey states in his *Food, Sex and Strangers*: 'It is possible that religion began as a kind of interspecies etiquette – especially when members of one species needed to eat members of another' (2013: 2). Religions have regulated food issues, either because of the heavy weight of tradition that tends to determine what people treat as significant, or because we perform our everyday activities, such as eating, in a religious manner (Harvey 2013; 2015). Religion has everything to do with the relationships that constitute, form and enliven people in everyday activities in this material world. Even for an atheist, Sunday lunch with family can be 'sacred'. Believing or not, we attribute 'religious' specialness to things and act accordingly. Hence, religion, in a wide sense, has shaped eating habits, therefore taste.

As a culinary art teacher I have had the opportunity to closely observe people's food choices for many years. I conclude that religion is an important filter, even for people or groups who declare themselves to be atheists or agnostics. Indeed, this fact made me want to study religion so that I could better understand the motivation for food choices. Moreover, having spent twelve years as a practitioner of Candomblé, I can affirm that food practices can reinforce religious adherence.

In this chapter I will show how food practices within a religion constitute a *food language* and therefore how religions can be professed through matters of taste. As a theoretical approach, I follow Lévi-Strauss' ideas in *The Raw and the Cooked* (2010a) in which he demonstrates that food rules work like any language. People's values and thoughts are expressed the same way, following the same rules, whether they are using verbal language or communicating through food. I also follow Mary Douglas in 'Deciphering a Meal' (1997) in order to demonstrate how meals follow a structure which encodes messages. I will exemplify these ideas by exploring the food practices of Candomblé, a religion based on the cult of African deities. Like other religions, Candomblé has its own taste, which originated in combinations of specific meaningful ingredients, most of which are mentioned in its myths.

In this chapter I will focus on Brazilian Candomblé. Because Brazil was colonised by the Portuguese, Candomblé and other African religions practised there have a Portuguese touch. This is demonstrated not only by the use of Portuguese orthography for Yoruba liturgical words, but more significantly by the food offered to the deities. For example, some of the typical ingredients or techniques of African votive dishes were substituted by Portuguese ones. The chapter first provides some background context, and then describes Candomblé's food practices and rituals. The final part of the chapter is more analytical, examining Candomblé's food practices through language theory.

CONTEXTUALIZING RITUALS IN AFRICAN AMERICAN RELIGIONS

The African diaspora in the Americas produced several interrelated religions, all of which are based on the cults of African deities. Cuban Santeria, Haitian Vodou, Surinamean Winti and Brazilian Candomblé, Xangô and Tambor de Mina are some examples. Some African groups managed to preserve their ancestral beliefs and some of their religious practices (Parés 2006). However, these African diaspora religions incorporated many elements from European Catholicism, and sometimes absorbed native American influences as well. Many of the deities worshipped in these traditions seem to be quite similar, and the ways in which they are worshipped have many common elements, such as the use of food offerings as a means of communication.

The cults focused on in this chapter all originated among the Yoruba of what is now Nigeria. The deities are called *orisas* (in Yoruba), *orishas* (in Spanish-speaking countries) or *orixás* (in Portuguese-speaking countries). In Latin countries they are also known as *santos* (saints). Each *orisa* represents, or is itself, a nature force to be venerated. They are worshipped by men and women by singing, dancing, obeying and by offering gifts, sacrifices and foods. Food offerings in African religions follow the idea of reciprocity, as says a Brazilian Candomblé ditty recorded by Vilson de Sousa Jr.: 'That who gives me to eat also eats, that who gives me to drink also drinks' (2009: 34)

Ancestors also play a very important role in Yoruba-derived religion. Just like the *orisas*, they are worshipped and never forgotten. They also receive offerings, some made by the whole community and some made by a single member or a single family. These offerings can consist of candles, leaves, flowers, objects, animals, drinks and foods. The foods offered could range from a single fruit to a whole meal prepared with the meat of a slaughtered animal. Collective offerings happen at specific times of the year according to a liturgical calendar. Individual ones such as rites of passage or healing rituals do not have fixed dates but are determined by circumstances. In all cases, the goal is to produce, transfer, accumulate, activate or expand the what is called *ase*, *ashé* or *axé* (in Yoruba, Spanish and Portuguese respectively) which consists of a force that animates all living things and moves the whole universe, according to Yoruba cosmovision. Another concept shared by several African American religions is *Ifá*, a set of poems or myths from which derive all the principles of such religions. Although it is orally transmitted, it can be considered the 'sacred book' of African-American religions as the African philosopher Kólá Abímbólá states (2006: 47). *Axé* and *Ifá* will be discussed in more detail in the following section.

CANDOMBLÉ, A FOOD-RELIGION

Food is a simple and familiar reference, recognisable by everyone, and therefore provides material for excellent metaphors, or even metonymies

Candomblé's Eating Myths

in which a food can actually be a part of an entity instead of merely representing it. Beyond symbolism, food issues can be so central in some religions that we could classify them as *food-dependent religions* (meaning that they would be very different without food practices). Candomblé exemplifies this model.

Ifá, the origin of everything

Candomblé mentions food, eating, offerings and related matters throughout *Ifá*, its sacred canon. All wisdom and principles of traditional Yoruba people are contained within a collection of 256 oral myths or poems – *itan* (story) or *odu* (destiny, path). Each *itan* tells a myth from which it is possible to divine the kind of destiny (*odu*) a person was born with and what might be done to ease it. *Ifá* priest Fá'lókun (1992: v) states that *odus* represent the energy patterns that create consciousness, analogous to Carl Jung's archetypes, i.e. each person shows features under the *odu* they were born. A person's *odu* is revealed through a divination system using palm tree seeds (*opele*) or cowry shells (*búzios*). In this sense, *ifá* is also an oracle (Figures 4.1 and 4.2).

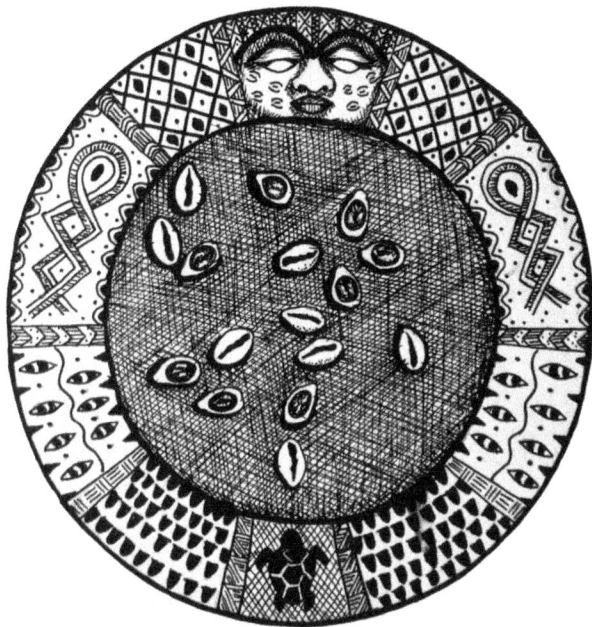

Figure 4.1 *Ifá* divination board with cowry shells. Drawing by Patricia Rodrigues de Souza.

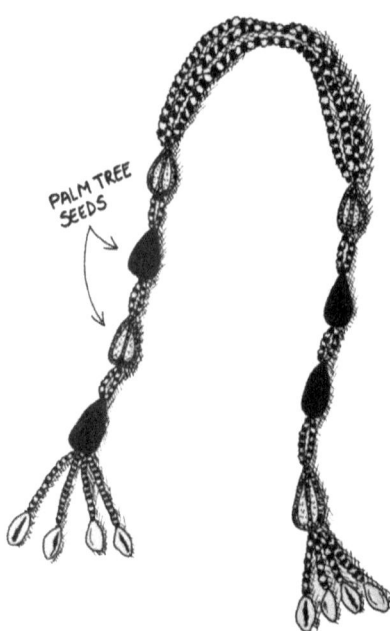

Figure 4.2 *Opele*, made with palm tree seeds. Drawing by Patricia Rodrigues de Souza.

In order to be animated, both *opele* and *búzios* must 'be fed', i.e. be offered food, usually including the blood of a slaughtered animal. From time to time they must be fed again to renew *axé*, the force that makes them animated and capable of communicating between priest/ess and deities.

Ítans contain the explanation of the context as well as indicating what religious procedures or rituals should be performed. They determine how offerings are made, to whom, by whom and when. For instance, when someone offers food to Xangô, they must also offer to his wife, Oxum, because there is an *ítan* that says they 'eat together'.

Ítans specify not only what should be used, but also those foods which are forbidden. A person who is going to be initiated will be told by the *Ifá* priest/ess (*babalorixá* or *ialorixá* respectively) what foods they are forbidden to consume after initiation. A common taboo for Candomblé's practitioners is scaleless fish. Some Candomblé practitioners have reported cases of people getting allergies or feeling sick when breaking a taboo (*ewó* in Yoruba, *quizila* in Portuguese). Also, some priest/ess will argue that when people have allergies or get sick from certain foods is because they are disrespecting a taboo without knowing it. Certain substances are not compatible with some *odus*. Most of the *quizilas* can only be discovered through

Ifá, but some are integral to a person's relationship to an *orixá*, e.g. those initiated to Oxóssi (the hunting god) cannot have honey. There is an *ítan* that tells how Oxóssi almost lost his son when the boy in the forest tried to get honey from a hive and got stung by several bees. Oxóssi swore never to have honey again. Not all ingredients used in Candomblé's food offerings appear in the *ítans*: ingredients introduced in the Americas are not mentioned, they are part of an adaptation process.

Axé, food for body and soul

In Candomblé's cosmovision everything needs to be nourished by what many insiders compare to a 'vital force', called *axé*. Brazilian scholar and Candomblé practitioner, José Beniste (2014: 278) defines *axé* as a magic fluid that has no shape but can be felt and gives life and shape to everything that exists. In its actions of creating and recreating, *axé* wears itself out and needs to be rekindled using precepts, foods, herbs, ditties and several rituals which will allow a constant relationship between the *Àyié* and the *Òrun*. *Àyié* is the material dimension where we live, while *Òrun* is the dimension where the deities, ancestors and our doubles or spiritual forms are. The emanations of food offerings, *axé*, are supposed to reach *Òrun* and therefore, feed *orixás* and ancestors. *Axé* circulates continuously between the two worlds in an eternal cycle, passing from one being to another, from plants to animals, then to deities and ancestors, then back to the soil. Brazilian anthropologist ethnologist and Candomblé practitioner Raul Lody (2004: 27) states that the main way to transmit *axé* is by offering food: to eat is to activate *axé* – energy and fundamental force – in Candomblé houses and people's religious lives. No matter if it is a person, a deity, an ancestor, an animal, a plant or an object, every being needs *axé*. Lody says

> the ground eats, the central mast eats, the gable eats, the door eats, the gates eat, the drums eat, the shrines eat, the trees eat. To eat is to make contact and to establish fundamental connections with the life, *axé* and the ancestral principles of the Candomblé house. (2004: 28)

FOOD RITUALS

Candomblé is a thoroughly ritualistic religion; the body is the main apparatus for spiritual actions (Beniste 2014: 219). There is no ceremony or initiation, collective or individual, where body practices do not play a prominent role. Food is associated with many of these practices. To illustrate this, I will describe two rituals, *Borí* (an individual feeding ceremony) and *Xirê* (a communitarian banquet).

Borí

Candomblé considers the head (*orí* in Yoruba) to be the most important part of the body. There is the physical head, *orí ode*, which supports all the rituals, and the *orí inu*, the head which comprehends the person's soul and which is affected by rituals. *Orí* connects the person and to his or her dominant *orixás*. Indeed, *orixá* means 'the owner of the head'. Every person in life will be devoted to and guided by his or her dominant *orixás*: as it is popularly said, a person is daughter or son of an *orixá*.

When a person is going to be initiated in Candomblé, the first thing to do is to strengthen his/her *orí*, the head, by feeding it. The procedure to do so, *Borí*, literally means 'to give food to the head'. The *Borí* will take place in a room attached to the Candomblé house, the *quarto de santo* (saints' room). During the ritual, the initiate is lain down, surrounded by several dishes containing the *orixás'* votive foods (Figure 4.3). Each *orixá* has its own dish and all *orixás* are offered food in this ceremony. A tiny bit of each food from each dish is put on the top of the novice's head and it is covered tightly by an *ojá* (ritual white head-cloth). The initiate will stay overnight in the *quarto de santo*, surrounded by all dishes containing the *orixás'* food as well as the food on top of his/her head. The initiate is not allowed to stand up or leave the room, except for a toilet break. S/he can eat as much as s/he wants from the surrounding dishes using only her/his hands; cutlery is not allowed in the *quarto de santo*. Priests and priestesses, as well as family members, are also allowed to eat from the surrounding dishes when they go for the ceremony. The surrounding foods are supposedly 'magnetised' with *axé*. The initiate will stay confined from three to twenty-one days, depending on the *Borí*'s goal. Other foods, different from the surrounding dishes, will be delivered to her/him three or four times a day, but such foods also follow precepts – during this process the initiate is not allowed to eat many other things. It is a sort of fast, not in terms of quantity (there is no limit to eating) but of quality, i.e. of ingredients. After such days, the initiate is permitted to leave. The leftovers of the food offerings are always dispatched in specific places, such as sea, forest, river, cemetery or crossroads, depending on the deity to whom it was offered, e.g. if it was offered to Iemanjá (the sea goddess), then it will be taken to the sea.

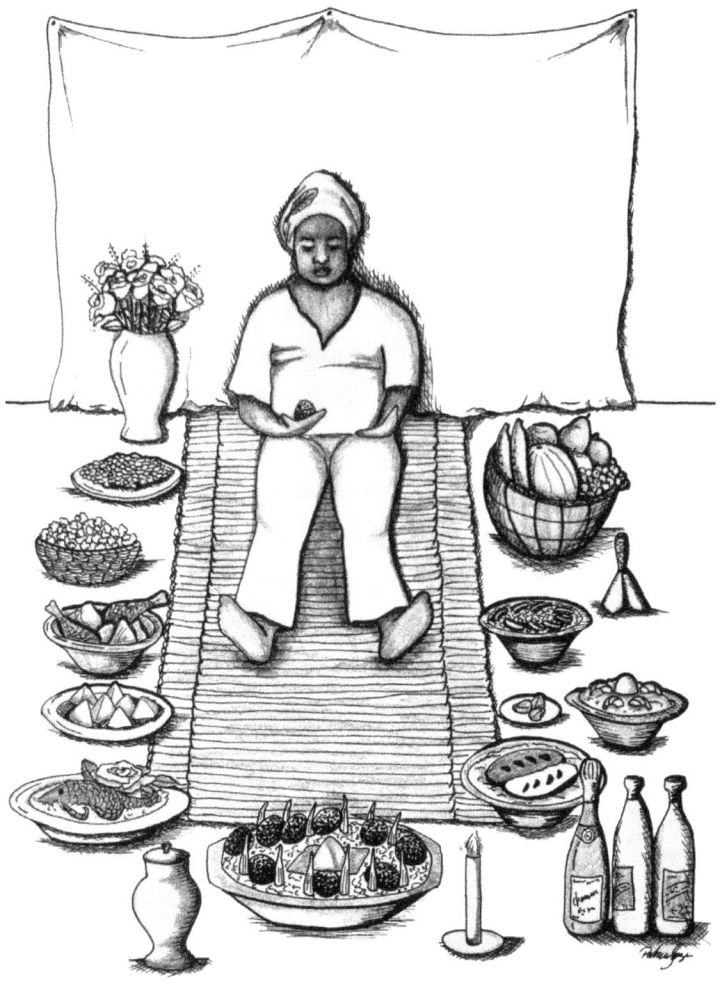

Figure 4.3 *Borí* ritual: initiate surrounded by votive foods. Drawing by Patricia Rodrigues de Souza.

Xirê

All year round, devotees of Candomblé pay homage to the *orixás*. In every communal ceremony (*xirê*) a different *orixá* is worshiped, according to the *ifá*. Each event in Candomblé's calendar is frequently remembered by its flavour, because in each *xirê* the votive food of the worshiped *orixá* is served to everybody.

Xirê is a huge banquet that takes place in the biggest salon of the Candomblé house. The preparations start early in the morning when an animal related to the honoured *orixá* is slaughtered and prepared in accordance to the precepts. Blood and offal are set apart because they cannot be consumed by humans. Blood goes partly to the soil and partly to the *orixá*'s shrine. Offal is taken to the Candomblé house's kitchen where it is seasoned, cooked and carefully displayed on a clay or wooden plate and placed in front of the *orixá*'s shrine. The carcass and meat are also seasoned, cooked and displayed on another clay plate; they are supposed to be impregnated with *axé* from the honoured *orixá*. These foods ought to be consumed by the priests, priestesses and other Candomblé house members, so they get *axé* reinvigorated. Other foods that meet the honoured *orixá*'s taste are prepared in the kitchen and served together.

In the afternoon, the main salon of the Candomblé house is nicely decorated using honoured *orixá*'s colours and symbols. The same sort of votive food served to the honoured *orixá* is prepared now in large quantities to serve the whole community and other guests at the banquet that will take place from the evening throughout the night. It feels a lot like a party. People dress either in their *orixá*'s colour or in the honoured *orixá*'s colour. Drums are played vigorously, loudly calling for all other *orixás* who come to possess their 'horses' or mediums (who may be either male or female). There is a sequence of the *orixás*' ritual dances, where myths from *Ifá* are retold in form of body language. As the dances take place, food prepared in the afternoon and drinks (usually soda, fruit juice and champagne or beer depending on the honoured *orixá*) are served in the salon; guests eat sitting or standing. Everyone person gets a plate filled up with food, indicating prosperity. Candomblé priestess Mãe Stella de Oxóssi says:

> the dynamics of eating and drinking in Candomblé transcend the biological action and constitute the main means to renovate and establish *axé*, everything starts in the kitchen and nothing can be compared to the energy that emanates from the offerings to the *Orixás*. Right after the offering ritual, *axé* expands through the rooms, ceremony hall, houses and city. (quoted in Lody 2004: 17)

IABASSÊ: ORIXÁS' CHEF DE CUISINE

The preparation of ritual food is so important and complex that it requires a special position. A priestess named *Iabassê* (always a woman) is the person responsible for all the work involving animal sacrifice, food preparation and serving *orixás*. A priest (always a man) named *Axogun* slaughters the animal but after that all preparation is the *Iabassê*'s job. Usually *Iabassês* are older and skilful women: they must know cooking, sewing, decorating, fixing. It takes many years to form an *Iabassê*, they start young as helpers, but will be only be initiated when they are older. One cannot choose oneself to be an *Iabassê*, some women are born to be so but must be identified by the *Ifá* oracle. The challenges of Candomblé's kitchen go beyond mastering cooking techniques: the *Iabassê* must know how to prepare a dish from skinning to cooking an animal. She must know each *orixá*'s foods, how they should be served and on what occasion. When several *orixás* are going to eat there is a precise sequence for the dishes to be prepared and served. Different dishes are served in different plates. Other than preparing *orixás*' food offerings *Iabassês* are supposed to know how to dress the *orixás*, and interpret their signs (they communicate only by subtle gestures). *Iabassês* do not get possessed for they are the keepers of *orixás* and of the mediums possessed during ceremonies.

At a Candomblé house, the kitchen is the domain of the *Iabassê* and is considered a special or sacred place where only ritual food can be prepared. When the *orixás*' food is being prepared either the *Iabassês* sing to the *orixás* or they remain silent. According to the Brazilian anthropologist and Candomblé practitioner Vilson de Sousa Jr.,

> In the kitchen we learn not only the proper consistency of dishes, but also that one should never turn back on fire, never throw salt on the ground, that the only spoons allowed to touch the food are the wooden ones, that food stirred by two people turns out bad – everything that happens in the kitchen assumes a special meaning: a knife that falls, small burns or cuts, food that burns or gets rotten are interpreted as signs, as if the *orixás* would speak through such gestures. (2009: 69)

CANDOMBLÉ'S SHOPPING LIST

The menu of offerings was originally made only with what existed in Africa before colonisation and slavery. However, this varied because Africans came from places with different ecologies, habits and cultures. Sometimes it is also very difficult to trace one ingredient's origin. In the case of black-eyed beans, for example, some authors will say it is African and some will say it is Asian. A few ingredients are surely African emblems – palm oil, okra and yam – and they are mentioned in the *Ifá*.

According to Bahian food specialist Guilherme Radel (2006: 51) yams carried from Africa their religious and agricultural significance: from the very beginning of African religious manifestations the liturgical calendar started with the harvest of the new yams, associated with the West African agricultural cycle. Juana Elbein dos Santos (1986: 228) argues that palm oil is certainly the most emblematic ingredient. Added in sacrifices and food offerings it is considered a 'vegetal blood', potentially replete with *axé*. Brazilian food historian Luis Cascudo (2004: 166) emphasises the importance of game, because at the time of colonization animal husbandry was not common. Some foods from Asia reached Africa before colonisation, so that rice and coconut were already familiar to African slaves arriving in Brazil.

The Portuguese transplanted spices and sugarcane from India; beef, pork, chicken and wheat from Europe; tomatoes, corn, potatoes, manioc, cocoa, avocado, pineapples, peanuts from the Americas; and palm oil, okra and yams from Africa. Africans did not start using Brazilian native ingredients such as corn and manioc only when they arrived in Brazil as the Portuguese had taken some foods to grow in Africa to feed slaves while they waited (sometimes for months) to be taken to America. Eventually yam flour was substituted for manioc flour, and sorghum mush for corn mush. The Portuguese influenced African sacred cookery not primarily by introducing new European ingredients, but by introducing new cooking techniques. As Cascudo (2004: 167) records, there were no stews or Portuguese *esparregados*. Originally, Africans did not know frying or sautéing but only roasted or boiled meats.

CANDOMBLÉ'S MENUS

Although some culinary elements are pervasive and easily recognised, the process of adaptation to new environments, with their lack of some ingredients and the encounter with new cultures, means that in different Candomblé houses there are now different dishes for the same *orixás*. Even in Candomblé houses located in the same city, within the same cultural/economic environment, dissimilarities in ingredients, preparation or decoration are found. The menu presented here is not a single homogenised pattern. I have considered my own experience as an *Iabassê* in a Candomblé house in Sao Paulo and *Santo também come* (2004; *Saints also eat*) by Lody, who compared votive foods in Bahia and Recife. I have chosen the most common ones, those which appear in more than three places. Moreover, within the sources above not all *orixás* are mentioned, only those most commonly worshipped and/or best known.

There are mainly two types of food in Candomblé's offerings: dry (made with vegetables and/or legumes) and wet (made with the meat of slaughtered animals). Although a person is free to offer either one as a gift, usually a consultation with *Ifá* will determine what should be offered – and in case of slaughtering, which animal. However, there is a pre-knowledge of what are *orixás*' favourite foods.

One flavour that must be really stressed in Candomblé's cookery is the *tempero de axé* (*axé* seasoning). It is the seasoning for all *orixás*' foods and consists of a mixture of onion, dried shrimps and palm or olive oil which characterises Candomblé's taste.

Food sociologist Claude Fischler (1988: 284), using psychologist Paul Rozin's concept of *flavour-principles*, explains that 'certain olfactory and gustatory complexes typical of a given cuisine such as the garlic-tomato-olive oil complex of the Mediterranean cuisines, are markers, taste motifs, making a dish recognisable and therefore acceptable even if some the other ingredients are alien to the system'. Religions with dietary rules or considerable food practices, such as Candomblé, are likely to have *flavour-principles* just like any regional cuisine – in this case, *axé* seasoning. It must be made fresh by the *Iabassê*, and could never be bought readymade. Most *orixás*' dishes take palm oil, but those *orixás* related to the creation of the world, known as *orixás fufun* (white), take only 'white' food (majorly white, clear foods such as white corn, rice, yams, also pears, green apples). This dichotomy is a very important aspect of Candomblé and breaking it would be a taboo (*ewó* or *quizila*). Candomblé has clearly shown binary aspects, in Lévi-Strauss' sense (2010a), though instead of raw and cooked, to take or not to take palm oil is a food sign of the binary thought in Candomblé. The following menu starts with Exú's food and ends up with Oxalá's food, which also expresses a binary idea as Exú is the trickster, the nearest to humans, while Oxalá is the most celestial *orixá*.

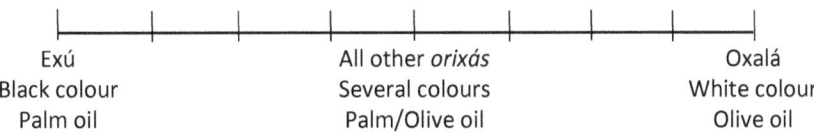

Exú	All other *orixás*	Oxalá
Black colour	Several colours	White colour
Palm oil	Palm/Olive oil	Olive oil

- Exú – always the first to be served because he takes the offerings to the *Orún*, the spiritual dimension where the *orixás* are. Without him no food is delivered. He is the lord of crossroads and frequently called trickster for his malicious way of doing things. One of his dishes is called *padê*. It takes toasted manioc flour with palm oil, adorned with chilli peppers. Raw meat can also be served to Exú, depending on the occasion and goal.
- Ogum – the *orixá* warrior. He is worshipped for helping in physical or symbolic battles. He is the owner of iron. Tools, knives, swords, anvils, lockers, railroads are attributed to him. Before preparing food, an *Iabassê* must ask Ogum's permission to use iron utensils in the kitchen. Ogum eats yams, those in phallic form, roasted, basted with palm oil. Another of his main dishes is black beans sautéed in *axé* seasoning. *Feijoada*, the famous Brazilian black bean and pork stew is associated with him. Many houses serve the *Feijoada de Ogum* (Ogum's *feijoada*) to all guests.
- Oxóssi – the hunting god. Arrows and bows are his symbols. His domain is the forest. He taught men hunting, though protecting pups and females. For that, he is associated with food and abundance, and with knowing how to get the necessities of life from the forest. Oxóssi's favourite dish is *axoxô*, cooked yellow corn grains sautéed in *axé* seasoning and adorned with coconut slices. Fruits are also much appreciated.
- Xangô – he is mentioned as the only *orixá* who used to be human and ascended to the condition of *orixá*. He used to be a king and still keeps this title as the king of justice. He carries two double axes that cut equally on both sides, thus representing impartiality. He is the god of thunderbolts, fire and stones. Okra is closely associated with Xangô, although it is also offered to other *orixás*. For each *orixá* okra is cut in a single different way; in dishes offered to Xangô, such as *amalá*, okra must be cut in strips, resembling a phallus shape, and then it is sautéed in *axé* seasoning. Many houses serve *amalá* with some meat stew, such as *rabada* (oxtail stew).
- Obaluaê – as the *orixá* that controls the world of the dead (*egun*) his domain is cemeteries and hospitals. He is also the called the doctor of the poor. Although slaves were precious merchandise, they were not treated by doctors, so when sick they would appeal to Obaluaê. Today Obaluaê is still a healer, compared to a shaman. His main food is popcorn, *deburu*. It must be made close to the time it will be used, and cannot ever be the microwave type. One *ítan* tells us that

Obaluaê had many wounds and could not walk in public. Feeling sorry for him, Iansã used her power over winds and transformed his wounds into popcorn and blew them away. Popcorn is therefore much used in healing rituals: people who are sick have their diseases washed away through a 'popcorn bath' (Figure 4.4).

- Iansã – holds a sword in one hand and a fan in the other. She is the goddess of war and fights along with Ogum. Her fan symbolises the wind controlled by her. She also shares with Xangô power over fire and thunderbolt. Her best known dish is *acarajé*, literally, 'edible fire ball', a dumpling made from black-eyed beans and fried in palm oil, gaining an attractive reddish colour. In Salvador, Bahia, many women sell *acarajé* on the streets. Most of these vendors are Iansã worshippers and they live by selling *acarajé* as a way to fulfil their destiny (as this is a way to worship Iansã). On their selling tray, there are always nine tiny *acarajés* that cannot be eaten because they are Iansã's. As she shares fire and thunderbolts with *Xangô*, she also eats *amalá,* Xangô's food, but her in her version okra is cut in slices instead of slivers.

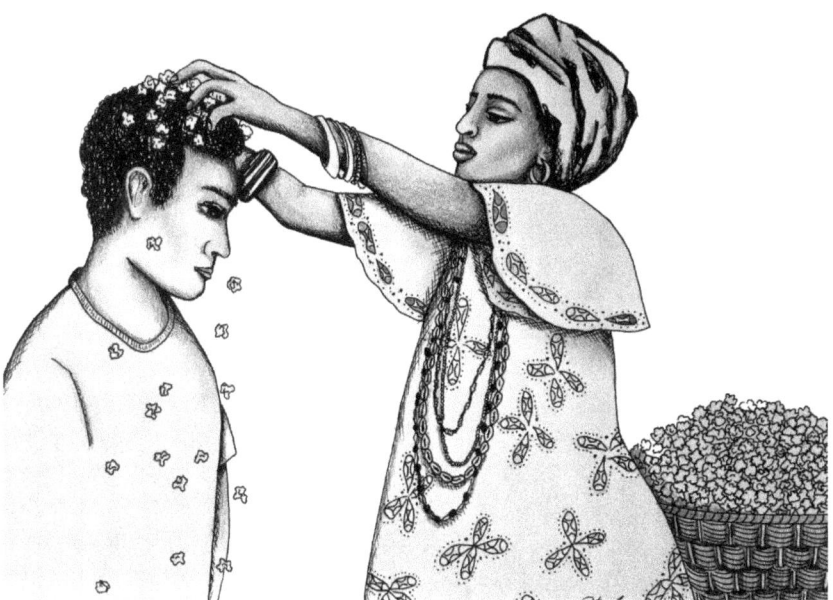

Figure 4.4 Candomblé priestess giving a devotee a popcorn bath. Drawing by Patricia Rodrigues de Souza.

- Iemanjá – perhaps the best-known female *orixá*, the goddess of the seas is very popular in Brazil. She is often represented as a mermaid. On 2 February each year, there is a huge procession to take Iemanjá offerings, usually foods and flowers. She is called the 'Mother of all heads', as she takes care of all *orí*. She is also associated with fertility, motherhood and families. According to African mythology she would protect slaves on the crossing of the Atlantic from Africa to Brazil. Her favourite dish is called *ebô*. It is made with white corn grains or rice sautéed in *axé* seasoning and adorned with fried shrimps. Iemanjá foods rarely have palm oil, but use olive oil instead because Iemanjá is Oxalá's wife and none of his foods can have palm oil. However, some households drop in a little palm oil because Iemanjá is Ogum's mother, and therefore she takes a little palm oil to join him. There's also a dessert, a coconut pudding called *manjar*, which is frequently offered.
- Oxum – her domain is the rivers and waterfalls; she is as sweet as river's water. Very sensual, she is the goddess of beauty, prosperity, fertility, pregnancy and small children. Being so graceful, Oxum had love affairs with Oxóssi, Xangô and Ogum. She is frequently appealed to in relation to fertility and love. Offerings asking for a mate or pregnancy are commonly adorned with yellow flowers and left by the waterfalls. Oxum likes *omolucum*, a dish made out of black-eyed beans sautéed in *axé* seasoning. Her offerings frequently include a hardboiled egg, representing fertility. Others of her foods include yellow fruits such as a kind of melon and a dessert called *quindim* (made from egg yolk and sugar).
- Nanã – the eldest female *orixá*, Nanã is wise and a sorceress. She controls rain and her domains are marshlands and cemeteries. As Obaluaê's mother she also manages the world of *egun*, the dead. She is so old that she is supposed to have provided the clay to create humans. One of her foods is *latipá*, black beans that have been individually peeled, by women only, and then cooked in *axé* seasoning. Another of her dishes is *benguê*, white corn porridge; in some houses it is sprinkled with a little sugar and cinnamon. She also likes sweet-potato balls.
- Ibeji – the twin *orixás*, representing children, a boy and a girl. The twins in the Yoruba system are associated with fertility, prosperity and joy. When someone gives birth to twins the whole community helps the family to raise them, as they are seen as a blessing. The

Ibeji's most common dish is called *caruru*, diced okra sautéed in *axé* seasoning. But they also get a tiny bit of every *orixá*'s food on their plate, representing the care given to children. Coconut desserts, candies, lollipops, fruits, honey and sweet tastes in general are highly appreciated by them.

- Oxalá – when several *orixás* eat and it is not a specific *xirê* for Oxalá, he is the last one to receive its food. This is not because he is less important but, on the contrary, because he is above the other *orixás*. He created the world before the *orixás* came. He is the *orixá* associated with peace, all his things are white, including his foods. Palm oil, salt or chilli peppers in his foods are taboo. Friday is his day of the week. On this day, in the old Candomblé houses nobody works, and nothing can be done that is associated with other *orixás*. Everybody wears white clothes and Oxalá's rice is served to the whole community at lunch time. Oxalá eats *acaçá* (a dough made from white corn, wrapped in banana leaves in the shape of a triangle), rice, white corn with coconut slices, and fruits such as green apples and pears which are considered white.

FOOD LANGUAGE

When we speak of Portuguese language, Spanish language or British language, we refer to a language as a cultural historical product, constituted as an ideal unit, recognised by the native speakers or by speakers of other languages and practiced by all integrating communities of such linguistic domain. (Bechara 2009: 37)

When we eat Portuguese, Spanish or British food, we refer to a cookery as a cultural historical product, constituted as an ideal unit, recognised by native eaters or by eaters of other cuisines, and practised by all communities utilizing culinary domains. Food historian Massimo Montanari (2008: 138) argues that each culture develops its food system (classifying, handling and consuming it) using conventions analogous to those which attribute sense and stability to verbal languages. Taste as flavour (sweet, salty, bitter or sour) and as value (good/bad) is a filter which implies classification and therefore meaning and symbolism. The culture of a society is symbolised in verbal language as it is in its foodways. The flavour-principals of a particular group's cookery are equivalent to the characteristic sounds (phonemes) of its language.

Food Grammar

The first important point of comparison between language and cookery (as a language) is the contrast between 'official' language/cookery and its variations. Modern language studies have increasingly considered language as something alive which changes, evolves and adapts. A language that does not show variations is a dead language. The same is true in cookery. When languages and ways of cooking are transplanted, they may influence the local language and cookery, and they may also be influenced by them. Grammatical structures may remain, yet new lexicons may be absorbed. Linguistically, this process is called lexical revitalization. Eventually and slowly, grammatical structure also changes, giving rise to either dialects or new languages.

Typical food and cooking practices of communities, even in religious contexts, may experience as many variations as languages. Lexical revitalisation is matched by 'ingredient revitalisation'. Such dynamics can explain many variations in Candomblé's food offerings. When *orixás* were originally worshipped in Africa, their food offerings would use only African local ingredients. After Candomblé was transplanted to Brazil, the cult of the *orixás* needed an 'ingredient revitalisation'. Not having the African ingredients available in the new land, people replaced them with local ones – e.g. millet was replaced by corn – just like when one language borrows a word from another. Not only the lexicon, but also the grammatical structure began to change: new cooking techniques such as sautéing (Portuguese *refogado*) started to be used along with the traditional African boiling and roasting.

As the African cults spread throughout Brazil, variations on food offerings multiplied, like dialects developing within languages. Today, every Candomblé house has its particularities and different identities expressed in their foodways. Lody (2004) has done extensive field research in Bahia and Recife, recording such variations. Despite all the changes something may remain unchangeable: okra is always present in Xangô's food, Obaluaê always gets popcorn, yams are Ogum's food, Oxalá will always eat white foods. They can be cooked, displayed differently or even mixed with other ingredients, but *flavour-principles* remain so that those dishes can be recognised as belonging to a particular *orixá*.

Going deeper into the relationship between food and language, Lévi-Strauss (2010b) says that cuisine (considering what is classed as eatable, ways of preparation and consumption, as well as the representations of digestion and elimination) come forward as a language in which each society codifies messages that allows it to signify at least part of itself. Lévi-Strauss has not only compared cuisine to language at the symbolic level, but explored the application of grammar rules to it as well, as he developed the concept of *gustemes* by analogy with the grammatical class of *morphemes*, minimal units of meaning in a language.

Morphemes can assume two main forms: *free* and *bound* as Trueba Andrade (2014: 11) shows: The word *unpredictable*, for example, can divided in three morphemes: UN-PREDICT-ABLE. PREDICT is a *free* morpheme in this word, since it consists of a core meaningful unit, whereas UN is a prefix denoting negation and ABLE is a suffix denoting 'can be done'. UN and ABLE alone are considered not to have real meaning on their own, therefore they are classified as *bound* morphemes. Free morphemes are semantically meaningful by themselves, while bound morphemes are grammatically, but not semantically, meaningful. Bound morphemes are intended to affect free morphemes' meanings.

Analogously, gustemes are the minimal gustatory units of meaning in *food language*. Gustemes can also be compared to Rozin's *flavour-principles*, mentioned above. As morphemes compose words, gustemes compose dishes. A gusteme can be a flavour of a single ingredient or a combination of ingredients that result in a single flavour, e.g. *axé* seasoning. As with morphemes, there are *free* gustemes and *bound* gustemes. Ingredients that can be eaten alone (such as beef), or are the main ingredient of a dish (such as lemon in lemon pie), serve as free gustemes. Ingredients that change the flavour of other ingredients and are not eaten by themselves are the bound gustemes, i.e. sauces, onions, salt and sugar. Ingredients are free or bound gustemes according to the way they are classified and consumed in cookeries.

In Candomblé's cookery, palm oil is a bound gusteme which denotes negation, due to the *orixás funfun* (explained previously): a dish that does not take palm oil designates a 'white' type of *orixá*. Oxum's *omolucum* will have black-eyed beans as the main ingredient and one of the possible symbols to represent Oxum – i.e. *axé* seasoning (onion + dried shrimp), and palm oil or olive oil depending on whether it is an Oxum of the *funfun* type or not. The dish *omolucum* is a 'word' formed by the gustemes oil (palm or olive), black-eyed beans and *axé* seasoning. Black-eyed beans are the free gusteme which gives semantical meaning to the word, whereas oil (palm or olive) and *axé* seasoning are bound gustemes which change the free gusteme, black-eyed beans.

The morpheme-gusteme analogy is summarised in the chart below.

Bound morpheme	Free morpheme	Bound morpheme
UN	PREDICT	ABLE
Bound gusteme	*Free gusteme*	*Bound gusteme*
PALM OIL or OLIVE OIL	BLACK-EYED BEANS	AXÉ SEASONING (onion+dried shrimp)

Just as morphemes together make words, so sets of words make sentences. Words ought to be semantically and syntactically related within a sentence to make sense. As ingredients have meanings, gustemes together make dishes and sets of dishes make a meal, but to make sense they must be prepared and served in a proper manner. In Mary Douglas' 'Deciphering a Meal' (1997: 36) there's an interesting dialogue in which two people argue about what to eat for supper. One of them suggests a 'good thick soup and after, to fill it up with a pudding' and the other answers this suggestion saying: 'What sort of meal is that? A beginning and an end and no middle!' A meal is never only a sum of selected and prepared ingredients; foods ought to make sense: roast beef is not a breakfast food, a coffee cake cannot be a wedding cake, barbecue is not proper for Christmas celebration, even though it is associated with celebration and most Christians are meat-eaters.

What and how (semantically and syntactically) foods are prepared and served in religious contexts such as Candomblé has an even more strict sense. It is not only a matter of eating in a way that makes sense, but it also implies a 'magical' procedure that aims a specific result. Offering the wrong substance, preparing it in a wrong manner or changing the order of serving it would mean to change the order of the world, which could bring disastrous consequences. It would not make any sense, and it could be offensive to offer Ibeji chilli peppers (which is Exú's food), or candies (Ibeji's food) to Exú. Also, Exú is always the first to get his food and Oxalá is the last to be served – also, his food cannot be 'contaminated' so everything must be clean before he is served.

The effects of semantic and syntactic changes are elucidated in the chart opposite.

Candomblé's Eating Myths

	SEMANTICS	
	LANGUAGE (English)	FOOD LANGUAGE (Candomblé)
Grammatically and Semantically Correct	I like dancing with my friends (verb)	Offering white corn grains to Oxalá
Grammatically and Semantically Incorrect	I *drink* dancing with my friends (verb)	Offering *yellow* corn grains to Oxalá

	SYNTAX	
	LANGUAGE (English)	FOOD LANGUAGE (Candomblé)
Grammatically and Syntactically Correct	I like dancing with my friends	Offering Exú first, then other *orixás* and Oxalá the last
Grammatically and Syntactically Incorrect	I dancing with my friends like	Offering any *orixá* before Exú

Meaningful ingredients combined in symbolic dishes, obeying the conventional order of preparation and service, make of meals full texts. Humans and other-than-human beings communicate through *food language*.

Metaphor or metonymy

Lévi-Strauss explained it perfectly when – in *The Raw and the Cooked Part III: The Fugue of the Five Senses* (2010a) – he compares myths to a fugue. That is, the same idea can be represented in different myths by different senses, as if expressions such as noisy, stinky, ugly, rough or bad taste symbolised the same occult meaning. Naturally, in this sense, these words can be understood as metaphors. Analogously, because foods are always attributed meanings, they can easily be used as metaphors. This is particularly observed in the religious context: Lydia Cabrera mentions honey as a well-known symbol of Oxum's sweetness (2004: 200). Okra, with its phallic shape resembles Xangô's masculinity (Reis 2010: 299). From the structuralist perspective, in Candomblé's *food language*, every *orixá*'s dish is a metaphor: a plate of *ebô* means Iemanjá, forces of the seas, etc. An *ebô* offered at the shrine will evoke a specific taste, colour, prayer, ditty, dance, stance.

From materialistic and/or theological perspectives, the *orixá*'s dishes are metonymy, a figure of speech consisting of the use of the name of one thing for that of which it is an attribute or with which it is associated, i.e. 'crown' for 'king'. Correspondingly, in Candomblé all foods offered to the *orixás* would be not a representation of them, but a physical part of them. Iemanjá, the sea and a *manjar* would be three different manifestations of the same type of *axé*. Similarly, Xangô, fire and *amalá* would be three different parts of another quality of *axé*. At the *Borí* ritual, because the novice is surrounded by all *orixás*' dishes, the *orixás* are present.

CONCLUSION

As Lody said in an interview in Brazil (2012), 'Food has so many functions that it's even good to eat!' Except in cases of extreme famine, humans never eat everything which is edible and neither do deities. If we ate only for nutritional purposes we would be now living on encapsulated food and religions would be then very different. It does not matter how digestible and absorbable substances are to the human body; they will be edible only when they are attributed meanings which make them 'fit' in the lived cultural context. At all times and in all cultures food taboos can easily be found, proving some foods are elected as not edible, either in declared religious contexts or in contexts considered secular. For example, foods such as meat, eggs, dairy or wheat may be treated as 'taboo' in such diverse contexts.

Humans have ideas about the goodness or badness of foods, in terms of their properties and tastes. But, as Montanari states, 'Food is not good nor bad by itself: someone taught us to recognise it so' (2008: 26). The taste organ is not the tongue, but the brain. Such a statement reinforces that foods taste like what they mean, and for most of human history religions have been determining not only what to believe and how to behave and dress but also what and how to eat.

In the northeast of Brazil, where Candomblé started, it is quite easy to observe the presence of African religion *flavour-principles* on daily menus. From the simplest to the most sophisticated houses, restaurants and streets of Bahia state, one can have *acarajé, caruru, omulucum, manjar, quindim* and an infinity of dishes spiced with palm oil, without even knowing these flavours are related to African religious cults. In the state's capital, the city of Salvador, there is a restaurant called *Iemanjá,* which serves many of the dishes that could be food offerings, but the people who eat there do not necessarily belong to Candomblé (de Souza 2015).

Naturally, we should consider individuals' agency. Nobody is an entirely sociocultural product, individuals may choose different religions, or different foods. However, there is always a background to our world view and it is possibly religious in some way. In ancient cultures or agricultural societies staple foods were commonly attributed to deities for them to nourish and keep many people alive. Because it was hard to obtain, food played a special role, and was valued for making gifts or for its central use in religious ceremonies and rituals. In our time, we are aware that food is still essential, but because it can be easily found, ready to consume, most people have lost, at least consciously, the understanding of how important and connected to life food is. Perhaps, this connection is manifested in the fact that there is something 'religious' in eating: the power of food to gather people together, the agency of food in the keeping of tradition and memory alive, food's property of embodying good values, etc. According to Fischler, 'Basic taxonomies incorporate the individual into the group, situate the whole group in relation to the universe and in turn incorporate it into the universe. They thus have a fundamentally religious dimension in the strict etymological sense of re-ligere, to bind together' (1988: 279).

Most of the time we think of taste as a matter of classifying something as having good or bad taste; in the best cases, we relate a certain taste to a memory; but we do not realize what structures taste implies and how this sense can give us information about ourselves and about what we believe. Eating presupposes beliefs. It is unlikely that a person would eat totally differently from the values s/he believes in. However, the meanings carried by foods and foodways help us to materialize our internal world when we choose to consume or avoid them, and especially when they are so significant that they are offered to special entities as gifts in exchange for beneficial outcomes.

REFERENCES

Abímbólá, K. 2006. *Yorùbá Culture: A Philosophical Account*. Birmingham: Ìrókó Academic Publishers.

Andrade, C. D. T. 2014. *Lexicon Across Borders: A Lexical Study on Trans-Lexicon Use in the Ecuadorian-Colombian Border Towns of Tulcan-Ipiales*. Doctoral thesis. Quito: Pontifical Catholic University. http://repositorio.puce.edu.ec/bitstream/handle/22000/10923/10.25.000059.pdf?sequence=4

Bechara, E. 2009. *Moderna Gramática Portuguesa*. Rio de Janeiro: Nova Fronteira.

Beniste, J. 2014. *Òrun - Àiyé. O encontro entre dois mundos. O Sistema de relacionamento Nagô-Yorubá entre o Céu e a Terra*. Rio de Janeiro: Bertrand Brasil.

Cabrera, L. 2004. *Iemanjá & Oxum. Iniciações, Ialorixás e Olorixás*. Sao Paulo: Editora Universidade de São Paulo.

Cascudo, L. C. 2004. *História da alimentação no Brasil*. Sao Paulo: Global.

de Sousa Jr., V. C. 2009. *O Banquete Sagrado. Notas sobre os de comer em terreiros de Candomblé*. Salvador: Atalho.
de Souza, P. R. 2015. 'Food in African Brazilian Candomblé', *Scripta Instituti Doneriani Aboensis* 26: 264–280. https://ojs.abo.fi/ojs/index.php/scripta/article/view/846 (accessed 13 June 2017)
dos Santos, J. E. 1986. *Os Nagô e a morte. Pàde, Àsèsè e o culto Égun na Bahia*. Petropolis: Vozes.
Douglas, M. 1997. 'Deciphering a Meal' in C. Counihan and P. V. Esterik (eds), *Food and Culture: A Reader*. New York, London: Routledge. pp. 36–53.
Fá'lókun Fatunmbi. 1992. *Awo, Ifá and the Theology of Orisha Divination*. New York: Original Publications.
Fischler, C. 1988. 'Food, Self and Identity', *Social Science Information* 27.2: 275–293. https://doi.org/10.1177/053901888027002005
Harvey, G. 2013. *Food, Sex and Strangers: Understanding Religion as Everyday Life*. New York: Routledge.
Harvey, G. 2015. 'Respectfully Eating or Not Eating: Putting Food at the Centre of Religious Study', *Scripta Instituti Doneriani Aboensis* 26 (Religion and Food): 32–46. http://ojs.abo.fi/index.php/scripta/article/view/849 (accessed 13 June 2017).
Lévi-Strauss, C. 2010a. *Mitológicas* – Vol. 1. *O cru e o cozido*. Sao Paulo: Cosac Naify.
Lévi-Strauss, C. 2010b. *Mitológicas* – Vol. 3. *A origem dos modos à mesa*. Sao Paulo: Cosac Naify.
Lody, R. 2004. *Santo também come*. Rio de Janeiro: Pallas.
Lody, R. 2012. Interview at Bienal do livro, Sao Paulo. https://www.youtube.com/watch?v=H6l9ypoWH5o
Montanari, M. 2008. *Comida como cultura*. Sao Paulo: Editora Senac São Paulo.
Parés, L. 2006. *A Formação do Candomblé. História e ritual da nação Jeje na Bahia*. Sao Paulo: Editora Unicamp.
Radel, G. 2006. *A Cozinha Africana da Bahia*. Salvador: Lei de incentivo à cultura/ Ministério da cultura.
Reis, A. M. 2010. *Candomblé : A panela do segredo*. Sao Paulo: Mandarim.

Patricia Rodrigues de Souza has been a Chef de cuisine and is currently a PhD student in religious studies at the Pontifical Catholic University of São Paulo, Brazil. She has taught Brazilian cookery and lectured on food studies. Patricia has observed religions, specially Brazilian Candomblé, through the lenses of food practices and has published a book in which she compares religions in terms of food practices: *Religion at the Table: A Sample of Religions and Their Food Practices* (Sao Paulo: Griot, 2015).

Section Three
SIGHT

Chapter 5
Sight and the Byzantine Icon

ANGELIKI LYMBEROPOULOU

This chapter addresses a very specific visual manifestation of Christianity, known as Byzantine art, the art of Orthodoxy. Orthodoxy was the official religion of the Byzantine Empire from 1054, following the schism that saw the emergence of the Orthodox and Catholic Churches. While the Byzantine Empire no longer exists, regions and lands that were directly under its control and/or influence still adhere to Orthodoxy (e.g. Greece, most of the Balkans, Russia and a large part of the population of the Central and Eastern European countries).

I start the chapter by looking at the role played by vision in Byzantine worship, focusing on icons. Then I consider the broader role of the senses in Orthodox veneration in the public space of a church, demonstrating how vision is intertwined with touch, hearing, smell and taste to enhance the experience of being in the presence of and revering the divine. I end the chapter by studying veneration in the private domestic sphere – focusing on a case study of an ivory scene, to highlight the 'multisensory' images in the presentation of different stages of the Gospels' narrative.

BYZANTINE ICONS

By far the most reproduced iconographic subject in Byzantine art is the Virgin and Child. Amongst the various reproductions the most famous and revered type is the so-called *Hodegetria* ('she who shows the way'). The name of the type relates to the place where the original icon was kept – in the monastery of the *Hodegoi* ('guides') in Constantinople. From the eleventh century onwards all sources invariably identify the *Hodegetria* icon

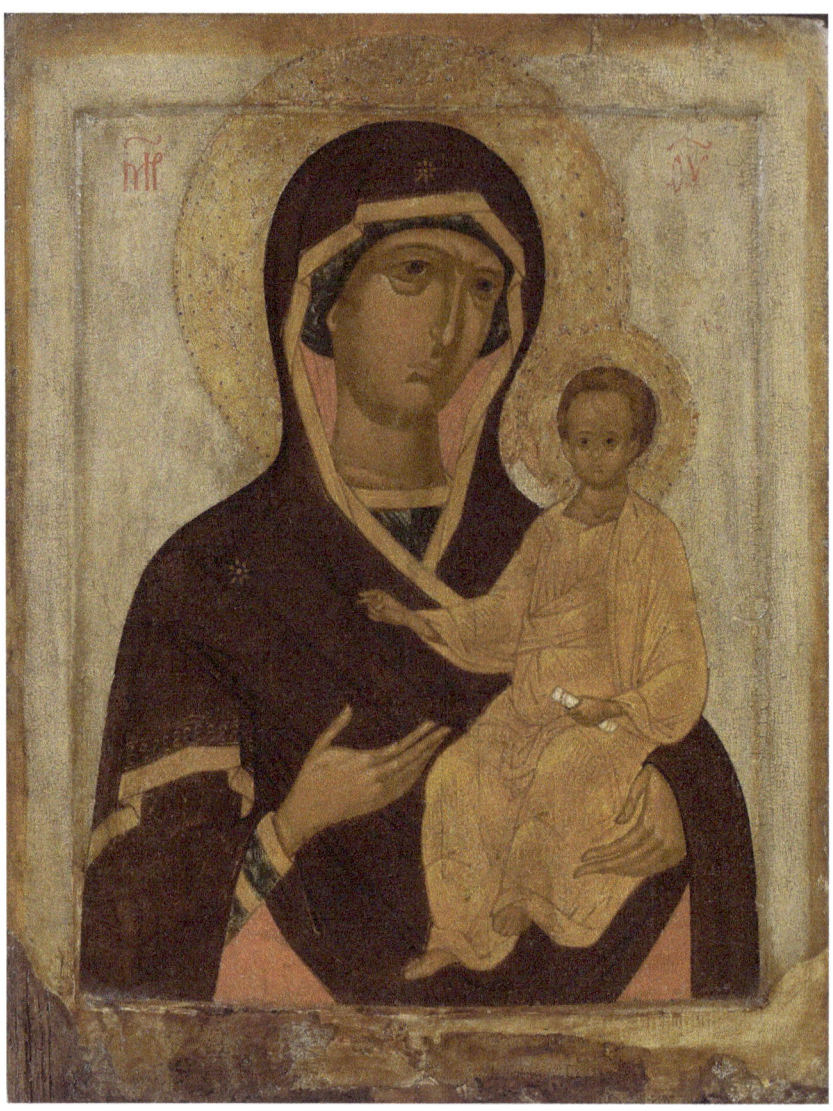

Figure 5.1 The Virgin *Hodegetria*, fifteenth century (?), panel painting, 58 x 46 cm, private collection. Photograph courtesy of AXIA-Yanni Petsopoulos.

found in the monastery with the *acheiropoietos* icon created by Saint Luke (a point to which we shall return). The icon was destroyed in 1453 when Constantinople fell to the Ottomans (Angelidi and Papamastorakis 2000: 378, 385; see also Woods 2013: 136 and n. 4). As is always the case with Byzantine art, it challenges sight to move beyond what meets the eye.

In the *Hodegetria* type the Virgin is depicted frontal and half-length (see Figure 5.1 for an example, now in a private collection). Her left arm, which is bent at the elbow, seems to support the Christ-Child, while she points at Him with her right hand. This is a very simple, two-dimensional, flat – one could even argue almost uninspiring – representation of the central figure of Christianity and His Mother. However, it would be wrong to dismiss it as such, for the icon, in all its simplicity, visualises a wealth of theological issues and acts as a window that opens up and invites us, through our sight, into a spiritual world. The flatness of the background helps towards achieving this goal, as well as the fact that it lacks any hint of physical surroundings – as viewers we simply do not know where the scene is set. It is also void of depth, suggesting that what we see is a divinity that neither resides in nor follows the laws of our natural world. We are, paradoxically, seeing the invisible. Turning to the Christ-Child, we might note that it is extremely difficult to ascertain His age. He is supposed to be a baby (certainly no more than a toddler), but He looks more like a miniature grown man. Closer observation reveals that His Mother's left arm, which we assume physically supports Him, actually does not. Christ effectively defies the most basic law of nature – gravity – and floats in the air. The icon thus prompts the faithful to comprehend that Christ may have a human form, but He is more spirit than flesh. This fundamental and crucial element of Christ's divinity is captured visually in this simple manner in which Byzantine icons of the Virgin and Child show Him being (not) supported by His Mother's arm. Finally, Mary with her free right hand points at Him; she puts Him on display for the faithful viewer. This visual indication of Christ resonates with the context of the original icon of the type, which was, as mentioned above, kept in the monastery of the Guides in Constantinople, whose main task was to show the way to others. The representation of the Virgin here thus underlines a fundamental precept of Christianity: that is, Christ is the one and only way that leads to salvation and eternal life. The Virgin Mary encapsulates this profound message with a very simple hand gesture. And while the viewers of this image observed the divine – depicted in a simple manner so rich in meaning – the divine figures themselves also observed the viewers, placing them under their auspices. In other words, while the invisible is seen it also watches and encompasses the viewers in its gaze.

Icons form the most characteristic religious 'trademark' of Orthodoxy – this is despite the prolonged and controversial debate within the Byzantine Empire known as Iconoclasm (literally 'the breaking of icons'), which started in the eighth century and ended in the ninth. Those opposing images, who were known as the iconoclasts, believed that there was no difference between Christian imagery and the representation of ancient Greek and Roman deities: in other words, these were two sides of the same coin, idolatry. The iconoclasts supported their objections with passages from the Bible, such as Exodus 20:4–5, Leviticus 16:1 and Deuteronomy 5:8 and 27:15, where the production of images is explicitly forbidden. Their opposition, the iconophiles (literally 'the friends of the icons'), believed that the devotion of each faithful viewer is not directed towards the material image, but rather to the actual saintly person and/or event it depicts. Their champion was the fourth-century bishop and theologian Saint Basil, who had stated that the 'honour given to the icon passes to the prototype', used as defence of the icons during Iconoclasm by Saint John of Damascus (c. 675–c. 749; see primarily Brubaker 1998; and also Acheimastou-Potamianou 1987: 37; Maguire 1996: 138; Evans 2004: 459 with n. 83). According to Saint John, 'everywhere we use our senses to produce an image of the Incarnate God himself and we sanctify the first of the senses (sight being the first of the senses), just as by words hearing is sanctified. For the image is a memorial' (Richardson, Woods and Franklin 2007: 364, with references to the original sources; see also Anderson 1980: 25). He thus pointed to our need for a visual 'vehicle' which could aid the human intellect to comprehend divinity, divine nature and divine environment – all concepts that are abstract, spiritual and do not follow the laws of nature.

At the end of Iconoclasm, the iconophiles emerged victorious and the succeeding period witnessed the steady rise of images in devotional contexts. The preferred medium for producing icons was painting, which enabled the Christian visualisation of divinity to distance itself from the three-dimensional sculpture that was so closely associated with ancient Greek and Roman religion. Over the years the word 'icon' has become practically synonymous to panel painting. It should be noted however that icons can be produced in any medium – wall painting, mosaic, manuscript, ceramic, stone, ivory, etc.

In his Foreword to this series, Graham Harvey states: 'For some people, this "doing of religion" is especially about cognition: the encouragement of correct believing or correct understanding.' One could argue that perhaps this principle lay at the heart of Iconoclasm. It is beyond the scope of this chapter to analyse Byzantine Iconoclasm considering past and present debates around the subject (Brubaker and Haldon 2011; see also Cunningham 2014). Nevertheless, regardless of where one might stand after such analysis, the fact remains that what we have come to identify as 'Iconoclasm' had a profound effect and lasting consequences on the presentation and appearance of Byzantine icons; in other words, its aftermath bears significantly on how they were visually perceived from the ninth century onwards.

By the end of Iconoclasm, Byzantine culture was in need of preventative measures against potential future controversies around the representation of divinity. Thus, in order to ensure that the devotion was passed to the actual saintly person and/or event depicted, as was fervently argued by the iconophiles, Byzantine artists tried to remain as faithful as possible to the very first iconographic representation for a particular person and/or event. It was felt that this close reproduction would ensure authenticity, as well as guarantee identification and safeguard against idolatry. However, it left little – if any – room for artistic imagination and innovation. Parenthetically, this is one of the main reasons why Byzantine art is often considered repetitive and unimaginative, a misconception about stylistic features which, in reality, has nothing to do with technical ineptitude of the artists, but can be traced to theological debates. The ability to visually identify images of saints and scenes was of vital importance for the Byzantines. Gregory Melissenos, the confessor of the emperor John VIII Palaiologos (1425–1448), while he was in Italy in 1438 to negotiate the union between the Orthodox and Catholic churches complained that 'When I enter a Latin church, I do not revere any images of saints that are there, because I do not recognise any of them' (Mango 1986: 254; Nelson 2007a: 102). The importance of a recognisable visual language, which effectively rendered the divine familiar and approachable, was at the core of the Byzantine icons' existence.

THE ROLE OF THE SENSES IN ORTHODOX VENERATION

Sources such as the tenth-century *Souda* lexicon suggest that Byzantine culture had a good grasp of the five senses. Its understanding relied on Aristotle's opinion expressed in his works on the senses (Περί Αἰσθήσεως καί αἰσθητῶν – *Peri Aisthiseos kai aisthiton* – which forms part of his work on the Soul – on which see James 2011: 13–14, with extensive references; see also Betancourt 2018), as well as on the work of the sixth-century philosopher John Philoponos. Under the entry for 'senses' (αἰσθήσεις – *aisthiseis*) in the *Souda*, sight is described as clearer (more distinct) than hearing; hearing clearer than smelling; and smelling clearer than either touch or taste (Brubaker 1998; James 2011: 14; see also Caseau 2016: 59; Nelson 2007b: 155). The fact that sight held such a prominent position in Byzantine thought (as reflected in sources like the *Souda* lexicon) may partly explain why the visuality of icons is of such paramount importance for Orthodox Christianity.

The first representation of any saint and/or event was considered as the 'prototype', the original that offered the rule of thumb for all subsequent reproductions. Moreover, to underline further the divine nature captured in original reproductions, some of them were classified as *acheiropoietes* (icons; singular *acheropoietos*), literally 'made without hands', implying that such images were produced with no human intervention, but instead either by saints or by miraculous acts. This is another vital point of Christianity distancing itself from pagan antiquity, by affirming that its divinity had a complete existence of its own and it was not created according to humanity's own image – a critique that was often made in relation to the Greek and Roman gods. Orthodoxy placed high value on its icons, which were considered miraculous, and the most important of them all was the Virgin *Hodegetria*, the type depicting the Virgin and Child discussed at the beginning of this chapter. It was believed that the original icon (the 'prototype') had been painted from life by the Evangelist Saint Luke himself; as such it was classified as an *acheropoietos*. It formed one of the main and strongest arguments for the use of images that the iconophiles presented, since it proved that reproducing 'likeness' had the approval of both Christ and His Mother; indeed, according to the narrative relating the episode, once Saint Luke showed the Virgin what he had produced, she said 'My grace shall be with this' (Angelidi and Papamastorakis 2000: 377; see also James 2016: 28–29). In the aftermath of Iconoclasm, on the one hand this functions as the ultimate approval of visual representation of the divine; on the other it sets this particular image as the rule that cannot and should not be sidestepped. Therefore, all subsequent reproductions and even slight variations that branched out from this essential core-type provided by the Virgin *Hodegetria* had to remain as close and as faithful as possible to what it depicted in order to maintain the all-important disassociation from idolatry.

Another *acheiropoietos* of crucial importance is the one depicting the *Mandylion* (Figure 5.2). Orthodox Christians believe that Christ made an imprint of His face on a cloth and sent it to the seriously ill King Abgar of Edessa (present-day Urfa in southeastern Turkey) who upon receiving it was subsequently cured of his disease (Cameron 1984; Guscin 2009: 141–159; Spanke 2000; Wolf et al. 2004; see also Spatharakis 2010: 340 and n. 226 [with extensive references]; Peers 2012; Bacci 2014). This story serves as a further justification for the existence of icons, since Christ Himself clearly

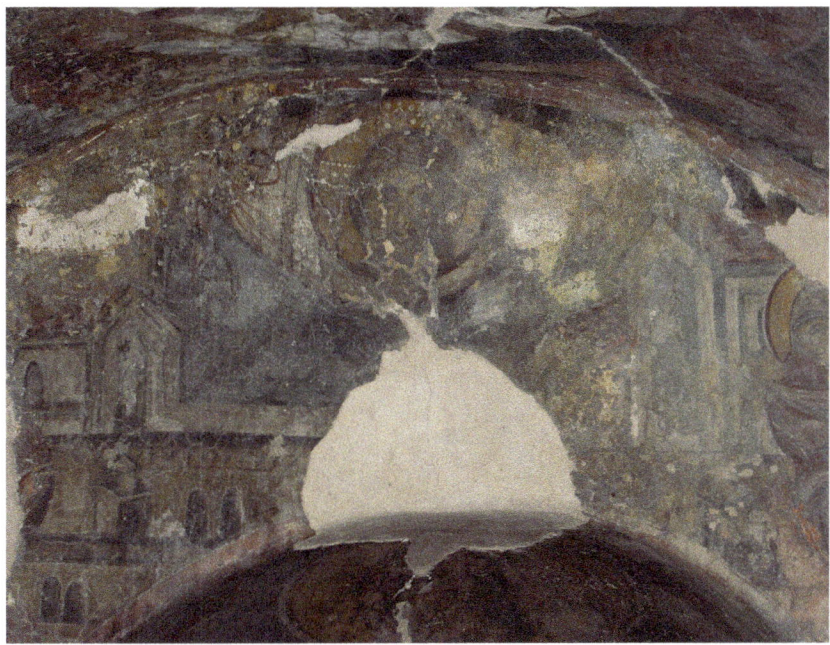

Figure 5.2 The *Mandylion*, 1319, wall painting, church of Saint George, village of Cheliana, prefecture of Rethymnon, central Crete, Greece. Photograph: Angeliki Lymberopoulou.

did not object to a reproduction of His likeness (Kuryluk 1991: 47–64). More importantly here, however, the story clearly suggests that there is strong relationship between Christ and His likeness, which could equally perform miracles since it is not a mere image of Christ – in some senses the *Mandylion is* Christ. Reproductions of the *Mandylion* are particularly popular as part of the iconographic programmes of Byzantine churches, the ultimate sacred space for any icon (it is important to remember that, as mentioned above, an 'icon' can be of any medium and size).

For Orthodox worshippers, icons can provide a door to a heavenly and spiritual domain irrespective of the space in which they are situated. In other words, they are capable of disseminating powerful and key messages, such as Christ being the one and only way, on their own. It is within the well-orchestrated space of the Orthodox Church, however, that they offer a more rounded illustration, within 'the earthly heaven in which the heavenly God dwells and moves' (Acheimastou-Potamianou 1987: 38). The architecture of Byzantine churches was interpreted as a representation of the visible and the invisible world, the spiritual world (Ćurčić and

Hadjitryphonos 2010: 99; note that the concept is applicable to all Christian architecture, and is not exclusively associated with Byzantine architecture). There is a variety of architectural types employed in Byzantine churches; the 'cross-in-square' or 'inscribed cross' with a dome, in use from the ninth century onwards, is one of the most popular and commonly associated with Orthodoxy. The 'hanging' architecture (a description that reflects the sensation that everything 'hangs' from the dome-heaven) with the *Dodekaorton* (from the Greek word δώδεκα - dodeka - for the number 12; a selection of twelve scenes associated with major events in the life of Christ based on the Gospels and Apocryphal narratives) at its heart, was first described as such by the Byzantine scholar Otto Demus in the middle of the twentieth century (Demus 1948). Over the decades it has certainly had its critics; it is true that Demus' analysis provides an oversimplified view of an extremely complicated world as presented in Byzantine architecture and its iconographic programmes. Having said that, it still provides a starting point for understanding key religious structures and functions translated in visual form within Byzantine Orthodoxy.

The basic rule of Byzantine architecture, whether a grandiose edifice with three aisles and a large dome, or a humble single-aisled tiny space with a barrel-vaulted roof, serving a village community, is that it offers the artists three well-defined zones where they can depict the hierarchy that prevails in Byzantine art and provides a visual vocabulary of key moments in the Orthodox calendar and liturgy, moving from top to bottom. Hence the top and highest zone stands for Heaven and it is here where Christ Pantokrator (All Ruler), the Virgin Mary, angels and the Ascension and Pentecost – scenes directly connected to Heaven – are depicted (in smaller-size churches that lack a dome, these scenes are represented in the conch of the sanctuary apse).

In the second zone, the faithful can see the narratives of the Gospels and the liturgy, including significant episodes from the life of Christ, representations of the Virgin Mary, and scenes from the life of the saint to whom the church is dedicated (for example, if a church is dedicated to Saint George, scenes from his life, miracles and martyrdom would be placed here). This zone represents Paradise. Significantly in the present context, in this zone we find a number of incidents in the life of Christ, which underline the importance of *visually* witnessing events in the matter of faith, but which also remind us how far these visions were originally intertwined with the other senses. For example, during the Baptism, Matthew (3:13–17), Mark (1:9–11) and Luke (3:21–22) describe the opening of the Heavens, the descent of the Holy Spirit in the form of a dove,

Sight and the Byzantine Icon 117

and the voice of God identifying Christ as His Son, while John (1:29–34) concentrates on John the Baptist bearing witness of Christ (seeing and hearing). Similarly, the centurion who often features in the Crucifixion is yet another witness of Christ's divine nature, since according to Matthew (27:54) he said 'Truly this was the Son of God' (seeing and hearing). The All Hail of the myrrh-bearers is another example where sight is aided by hearing, since this relates to the moment when the resurrected Christ met the two Marys on their way back from His empty tomb, and greeted them in order to emphasise His presence (Matthew 28:9).[1] In the Incredulity of Thomas, the disciple declared he would not believe that Christ was resurrected until 'I shall see in his hands the print of the nails, and put my finger into the print of the nails, and thrust my hand into his side' (John 20:25) (seeing and touching). Once Thomas was granted his request, Christ informed him that 'because thou hast seen me, thou hast believed; blessed are they that have not seen, and yet have believed' (John 20:29). However, it is evident in this instance that the persuasion of Thomas relied on a combination of seeing and touching, and that seeing alone would not have been enough. This same close connection between seeing and touching is found elsewhere in Orthodox religion, for instance in the kissing of the icons, a specific veneration that acts as a further confirmation that what the faithful see is the 'real thing', since they are able to touch (kiss) it. I would suggest that Christianity treats all faithful like Thomas and by shaping the abstract divinity in the form of an icon that can be seen and can be touched (Thomas' demand) nullifies the need for such requests.

The third and lowest zone is at the eye-level of the congregation and represents the terrestrial world. Here the faithful are surrounded by rows of individual male and female saints – martyrs, warriors, doctors, monks, stylites (saints who lived at the top of a column) and hermits. It is very difficult – if not impossible – to locate Orthodox churches with identical assemblies and presentations of saints in the lower parts of their edifices. In general it is difficult to locate any two Byzantine churches with the exact same iconographic scheme. While, however, the choices for the sanctuary, the place of the church closer to Heaven, are much more limited, and the choices for the second zone are dictated by the Gospels and the patron

---

1   The famous episode narrating the *Noli Me Tangere* (Touch Me Not) found in John 20:17, where Christ instructs Mary Magdalen not to touch Him, is primarily depicted on panel; unlike the scene of *Chairete* ('All Hail') it does not customarily form part of the iconographic programme of a church; see Lymberopoulou et al. (2011).

saint and/or event to which the church is dedicated, in the lower part of the nave the assembly of saints tends to reflect more local and social needs, the needs of the community served and its affiliation and devotion to particular saints, the ones that are watching over them to ensure the immortal souls of the congregation will reach Paradise. The worshippers are literally surrounded by an entourage of saints and are hence reminded that in order to join and proceed to Paradise and Heaven above they have to be good Christians. Hence the saints also serve as examples that confirm a place in Paradise is possible. Saints turn an abstract concept into an apt visual reality which the congregation are able to witness and sensually interact with (certainly by seeing and reaching out and touching). Even the wax of the candles that burn before the icons, the offering of the faithful to accompany their prayers, as Osborne has put it, transforms into visible smoke that rises to the ultimate destination, the Heaven above, aided by the watchful saints (Osborne 2003: 145).

In order to drive the concept that the Christian way of living this life will bear fruits in eternity, the west wall of some churches, where the exit is situated, often depicts gruesome and highly sensory visualisations of hell and punishments of sinners in the afterlife (e.g. extreme pain, unbearable heat and thirst, and bad smell of decaying bodies and boiling tar). In other words, once the faithful make their way out of the church at the end of the liturgy, leaving behind them the safe space among their protector saints, this is the last visual imprint that they will carry with them, horrific images of penalties that will serve as a constant wagging finger to help them keep away from sins and temptation (Figure 5.3) and instead stay as much as possible on the path chosen by the saints.

In what follows I refer to contemporary worship in the Orthodox Church. However, it should be noted here that Orthodox religious rituals have a very long and established presence in the life of the faithful. The practices that are still observed today among Orthodox monastic establishments, such as in Mount Athos, hark back centuries and the transition from the Byzantine to present times has witnessed very few groundbreaking changes – the discovery of electricity, for example, had understandably some impact on the interaction between artificial light and the buildings' surfaces.

The environment that Byzantine/Orthodox churches provide for the icon(s) to be viewed and worshipped plays a fundamental part in the faithful person's experience. As I hinted above, sight alone does not reflect the full sensual experience provided by the Orthodox rituals; vision relies on the stimulation of the other senses and they all work together in order to

Sight and the Byzantine Icon 119

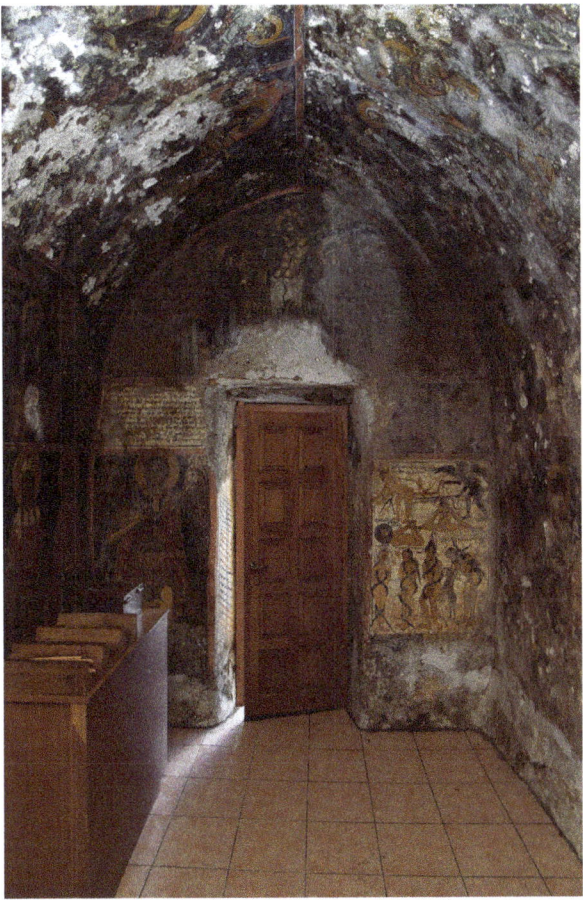

Figure 5.3 General internal view towards west of the church of Saint Paraskevi, 1372, village of Kitiros, prefecture of Chania, southwestern Crete, Greece: entrance/exit with wall painting depicting hell scenes. Photograph: Angeliki Lymberopoulou.

shape experience. The interplay of darkness and light is very important in Byzantine/Orthodox churches, regardless of their size, material and shape. Windows are normally small, and scattered around the church, allowing light to enter only at specific times of day. When natural light enters the church it often encounters the light provided by the candles burning before icons, which (as mentioned above) are often interpreted as visualising the prayers of the congregation carried by the smoke to Heaven. These two sources of light reflect on the building's surfaces (be they marble, mosaic, wall painting, wood) and animate the representations of sacred subjects.

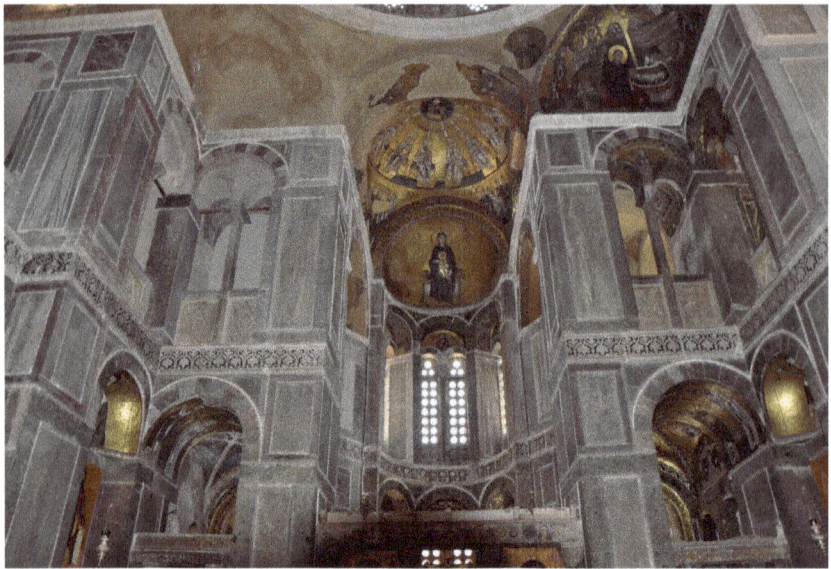

Figure 5.4 General interior view of the church of Hosios Loukas, eleventh century, Phokida, mainland Greece: detail with light reflecting on mosaic and marble decoration in the church. Photograph courtesy of the personal photographic archive of the late Dr Stavros Maderakis.

The depictions of the saintly persons and events acquire new dynamics of their own, propelled by the playful light (Figure 5.4).

Smell also plays an important role. Incense-burners are vital in Orthodox rituals: they can be free standing, hand-held or chain-mounted – the latter mostly used by priests in churches during the liturgy. At various times during the Orthodox liturgy, the priest would walk among the congregation with a chain-mounted incense-burner, the movement of which produces a very distinct and characteristic sound; members of the congregation are thus 'pre-warned' by the sense of hearing of the approaching incense-burner, and thus made alert to the smell. The combination of smell and vision (of the icons) forms a very strong link in this religious practice. Again, the intensity of such moments is always greater within the sacred space of a church; however, we should not forget that (primarily hand-held) incense-burners were – and are still – used in Orthodox homes (Cormack and Vassilaki 2008: 196–201 and 43 n. 217).

For those attending an Orthodox liturgy the sense of hearing is stimulated from the beginning to the end in a manner rivalled only by sight (Pentcheva 2010; 2011; see also Brajović and Erdeljan 2015). An integral part of Orthodox religious ritual is the chanting of hymns, based on Byzantine music, still presently in use within the Eastern Orthodox rite (Kazhdan 1991: 1424–1426). The senses are constantly challenged and work together in order to enable the congregation to 'see the invisible': the sight of icons, with their surfaces caressed by light, brings them to life and alludes to the fact that Christ is indeed the light of the world (John 8:12), mingled with the smell of incense against a soundscape filled with Byzantine music (Louth 2016). This in an environment where the congregation is also encouraged to kiss icons (Brubaker 2006) upon entering the church which allows the sense of touch to join in the experience. Even taste becomes involved when the faithful receive the Holy Communion, the Body and Blood of Christ from a cup in the form of a spoonful of sweet wine with a tiny morsel of bread.

The whole image is perfectly conveyed by the account of the Russian delegation that visited Constantinople in the late tenth century, offered to their prince Vladimir upon their return to their home country. When they entered Hagia Sophia they

> knew not whether we were in Heaven or on Earth. For on Earth there is no such splendour or such beauty, and we are at a loss how to describe it. We only knew that God dwells there among men, and their service is fairer than the ceremonies of other nations. For we cannot forget that beauty. Every man, after tasting something sweet, is afterward unwilling to accept that which is bitter, and therefore, we cannot dwell longer here [i.e. in Russia]. (Cross 1930: 199; Cross and Sherbowitz-Wetzor 1953: 111)

Parenthetically, it is very interesting to note that the delegation by being 'at a loss how to describe' the surrounding beauty, chose in the end to refer to taste in order to convey their powerful sensual experience.

A 'MULTISENSORY' IMAGE

So far we have engaged with the veneration of icons in public sacred space, carefully orchestrated and framed within rituals that stimulate all the senses in order to achieve the presentation of the divine to the faithful. But how does this work within the private context of a believer's household? Do the privately owned icons equally engage the senses? The first thing we need to keep in mind is that Byzantine iconography, by staying close to its prototypes, created a visually literate congregation that could, should and would have been able to recognise the key stages

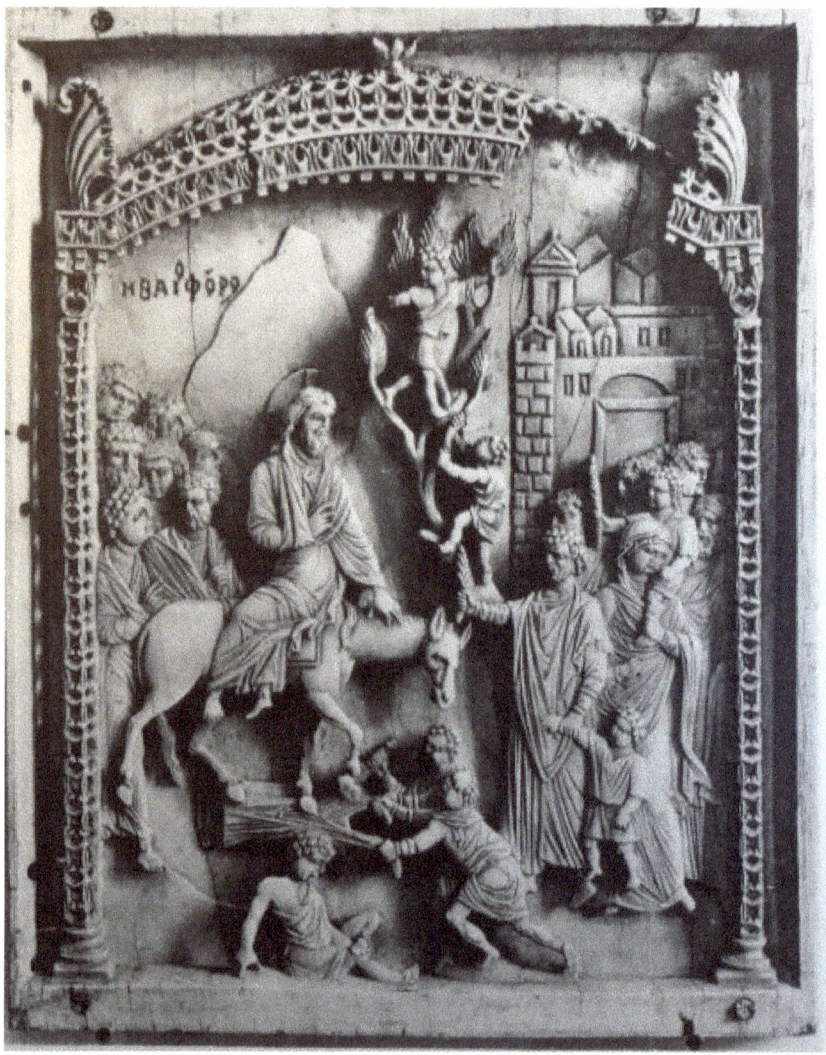

Figure 5.5 The Entry into Jerusalem, eleventh century (?), ivory, 18.4 x 14.7 cm, Museum für Spätantike und Byzantinische Kunst, Berlin, Germany. Photograph reproduced from Adolph Goldschmidt and Kurt Weitzmann, *Die byzantinischen Elfenbeinskulpturen des X.-XIII. Jahrhunderts* [2 vols, Berlin, 1934], vol. 2, Plate 3.

of Orthodox liturgy also independently, without the help of the Orthodox priest in the church.

For an example, we might look at the magnificent ivory icon currently in the Museum für Spätantike und Byzantinische Kunst in Berlin (Figure

5.5). The small dimensions of this object imply private ownership, while its craftsmanship and expensive material point to an affluent individual; the holes to the left side of its frame suggest that this was probably part of a diptych (two panels attached together); the inscription in Greek that identifies the scene in capital letters at the top left (Η ΒΑΙΟΦΟΡΟ – I VAIOFORO – literally, the bearing of palm branches) with correct spelling is indicative that the owner (who may have advised the artist) was educated. The ivory is traditionally dated to the tenth century, but a later date in the second half of the eleventh century is possible. Either way, it is a product of the Middle Byzantine period, the era that historically lasted between the end of Iconoclasm in 843 and the fall of Constantinople to the troops of the Fourth Crusade in 1204.

The Entry into Jerusalem is one of the pivotal moments in the life of Christ, because it signposts the beginning of His Passion, without which there would be no salvation for mankind. This episode is narrated by all four Evangelists: Matthew 21:1–9; Mark 11:1–10; Luke 19:29–40; John 12:12–15. Hence the individual would have been familiar through the Gospel narratives with a number of iconographic elements that the icon presents before their eyes: Christ riding on a donkey and about to enter the city of Jerusalem; the group of disciples who accompany Him and follow immediately behind; the mountain, rendered as a simple outline here, behind Christ and His disciples; and the group of people depicted standing outside the walls of Jerusalem welcoming Christ into their city.

The latter two – the mountain and the people – act as further visual references to the Gospel narrative: the mountain stands for the Mount of Olives mentioned in Matthew 21:1; Mark 11:1; and Luke 19:29 and 37. It reminds the faithful that it was there that Christ fully accepted that He should go through pain and suffering in order to save mankind. Had He refused to carry out the will of God (His Father), there could not have been any salvation. The crowd represent the Jewish people who according to Matthew 21:8–9, Mark 11:8–10, Luke 19:39 and John 12:12–13 came outside their city's walls to greet Christ. However, the four Gospels do not account for all the details that appear in the Byzantine iconography of this scene.

For example, the Gospels do not mention the two boys who are climbing up the tree in order to cut branches (a reference to the Greek title of the scene, 'bearing palm branches'), or to the children who spread clothes on the road, or finally to the boy in the foreground – a clear visual reference to a very popular statue from antiquity known as the *spinario* (thorn-puller). In an image aimed at helping the faithful visualise the Gospel narrative, what was the purpose of including elements that are not included in the Gospels?

While no children are mentioned in the four Gospels' narrative of this scene, they do feature in the Apocryphal Gospel of Nicodemus. This text was produced sometime in the fifth century and while it did not form part of the official church liturgy, it was nevertheless very popular and widespread among the faithful, and as a consequence had an impact on Byzantine iconography.[2] Furthermore, the children here probably offer a visual reflection of contemporary practices in the re-enactment of the scene during liturgical processions, an important aid in collapsing time between that of Christ and that of the contemporary faithful. Hence, through sight the other senses that would have been stimulated in actual processions are invited to jog the faithful's memory and remind him/her of the crowding and the closeness between people in such circumstances; the noise and murmur, which also references church chanting; the smells – including that of the fresh palms so pivotal in the celebration of this feast day. The owner of the ivory may have burned an oil lamp before it (Cormack and Vassilaki 2008: 434–435, cat. nos. 218–220; Petsopoulos 2016: no. 16), the flickering light of which would have reinforced the illusion of the unrealistically 'flying' donkey, which in turn would have highlighted Christ's spiritual being (just like the Virgin *Hodegetria* does). Even when the owner of the icon reached out to kiss it, the uneven ivory surface would have evoked the 'complicated' experience of partaking in a big procession with pushing, pulling, tagging, talking, smelling – the latter sense further encouraged by the possibility of burning incense before it.

Still the most intriguing detail in this ivory icon is offered by the thorn-puller which, unlike all the aforementioned elements, is not always encountered in representations of the scene. It is clear that the sitting boy, who is trying to extract a thorn from his foot, is placed on the same axis as and immediately below Christ riding the donkey. While the *spinario* remained a popular subject in Medieval and Renaissance times (Bober and Rubinstein 2010: 254–256 n. 203; see also Mouriki 1970–1972), it was far from the only popular sculpture from antiquity. Why incorporate this specific visual reference from the pagan past (and it should be noted here that this particular image bears no religious attachments to this past) into Christian iconography?

Shortly after Christ's triumphal Entry into Jerusalem, He was arrested, tried and mocked, before He was crucified. Part of the mockery was the

---

2 For the text of the Gospel of Nicodemus, see James (1924: 97, I §3).

placement of a crown of thorns on Christ's head, with the crowd hailing Him as 'King of the Jews'. The Gospel narratives present very powerful images of this scene: Matthew 27:29; Mark 15:17–19; John 19:1–3. In fact this crown was among the relics kept in Constantinople that were removed from the city after its sack by the troops of the Fourth Crusade in 1204 and ended up in France's Saint Chappelle.[3] It is highly likely the *spinario* in

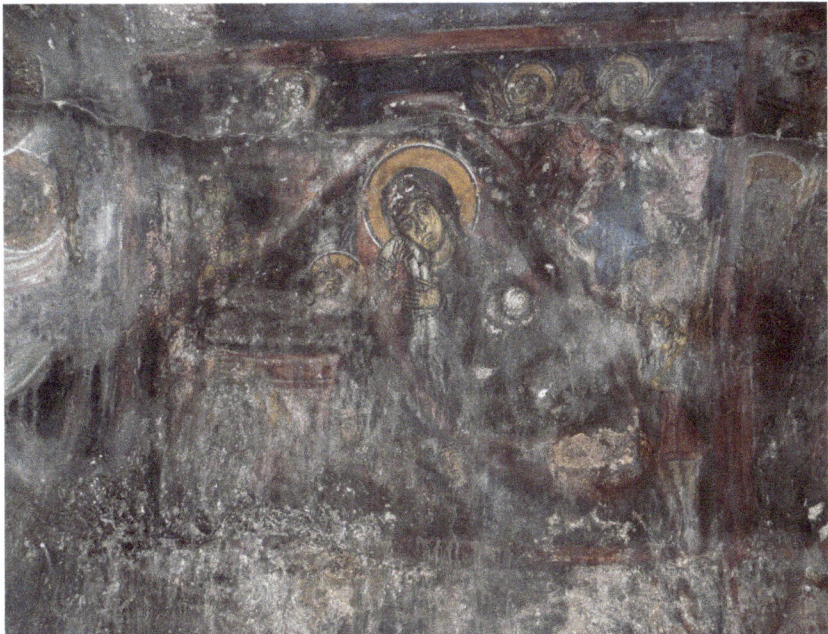

Figure 5.6 Nativity, fourteenth-century wall painting, Church of the Virgin of the Two Rocks, village of Fres, prefecture of Chania, western Crete, Greece. Photograph: Angeliki Lymberopoulou.

3 Cutler (1995, esp. 241). The crown of thorns was taken to Constantinople about 1063, where it was kept in the emperor's palace (Nickell 2007: 100–103). The cult of relics was extremely important in Byzantium (Hahn and Klein 2015). The ivory under consideration here is customarily dated to the tenth century; however the dating of a number of Byzantine ivories is neither secure nor undisputed. It is certainly beyond the scope of this paper to debate its dating; however, a date in the eleventh century and a direct connection to the arrival of the crown of thorns in Constantinople perhaps should be considered. Tony Eastmond has also raised the question whether the figure of the thorn-puller 'was added to give an extra layer of meaning to the image' (Eastmond 2013: 152).

this Constantinopolitan artefact with its prominent placement in the main axis of the scene and directly connected to Christ, the main protagonist, was deliberately put there as a strong, multisensory reference to what was to follow in Christ's life after this moment, namely His Passion with all the suffering, pain and the humiliation the crown of thorns represents. In other words, it is highly likely that this detail acts as a little symbolic glimpse into the future and encourages the viewer to think of what comes next.

Associative visual references are not uncommon in Byzantine art. While the *spinario* is probably indicative of a certain level of education, primarily of the ivory's patron, since it requires a level of knowledge of antique art, the majority of such references appeal to the wider congregation and do not require specific knowledge to decipher; they are rather meant to trigger the faithful's forward thinking in a much more straightforward manner. Such is the case, for example, in certain Nativity scenes where the Virgin is depicted holding to her cheek a piece of cloth (Figure 5.6). Christ's incarnation via His birth, as such a joyful moment, was one of many steps leading to the ultimate goal, His sacrifice through His Passion. Just as the Virgin was always aware of her son's destiny, the faithful should be too. Hence here the Virgin, via a tactile image of contact with cloth, is inviting the congregation to think thirty-three years ahead, to the moment when Christ's dead body will be lying ready for burial – an invitation further reinforced by the fact that the baby Jesus is lying horizontally to the right of the Virgin – as well as His subsequent resurrection. Therefore the cloth so prominently held by the Virgin is a visual reference to forthcoming events, all familiar to the viewer through the Gospel narrative: Christ's shroud in which He was buried as mentioned in Matthew 27:59 (clean linen cloth), Mark 16:46 (fine linen), Luke 24:53 (linen), and John 19:40 (linen clothes); and Christ's empty shroud as discovered by two of His disciples that marks His resurrection, narrated by John 20:5 ('and looking in, saw the linen clothes lying').[4]

---

4 In certain scenes depicting the Lamentation over Christ's dead body, a white sheet is sometimes placed on the stone on which Christ has been laid after the Deposition from the Cross (Lymberopoulou 2006: 80). This could be based in the Apocryphal Gospel of Nicodemus that describes the Lamentation and mentions a 'white sheet' (ἐν σινδόνι λευκῇ – en sindoni leuki) in which Christ was buried (Tischendorf 1959 [1853]: 291–292). It is possible that the cloth in the Virgin's hands in Nativity scenes, such as the one depicted in Figure 5.6, may also aim at providing an associative link to the Lamentation.

Giorgio Vasari, the sixteenth-century artist from Arezzo considered to be the first art historian, nurtured a very low opinion of Byzantine art and its (lack of) achievements. The Cretan artist Domenikos Theotokopoulos, better known as El Greco, contested Vasari's view: in the margins of his own copy of Vasari's *Lives of the Artists* (De Vere 1996), the Greek commented that Byzantine art is full of 'ingenious difficulties', and therefore not lacking skill (Hadjinicolaou 2008; see also Lymberopoulou 2007: 205-206 with n. 109). While El Greco does not elaborate on what these 'ingenious difficulties' may be, this chapter has demonstrated the complexity of the visuality of icons and the all-important need for them to reflect basic Orthodox theological positions. Icons lie at the core of Byzantine rituals and are expected to act as reference, and to stimulate and cooperate with all the other senses, aiming at providing the faithful with the complete Orthodox religious experience. Byzantine Art is at Orthodoxy's service and certainly Orthodoxy could not have been the same without its icons, a visual portal that leads all senses to another dimension. This chapter has demonstrated the subtle interrelation that sight weaves with other senses (for example touch), in order for Byzantine icons to enable the viewers to perceive, reach out and embrace the invisible divine.

REFERENCES

Acheimastou-Potamianou, M. (ed.) 1987. *From Byzantium to El Greco: Greek Frescoes and Icons.* London: Royal Academy of Arts.

Anderson, D. (transl.) 1980. *John of Damascus: On the Divine Images* 1, 17. Crestwood: St Vladimir's Seminary Press.

Angelidi, C., and Papamastorakis, T. 2000. 'The Veneration of the Virgin Hodegetria and the Hodegon Monastery' in M. Vassilaki (ed.), *Mother of God Representations of the Virgin in Byzantine Art.* Athens: Benaki Museum, and Milan: Skira editore. pp. 373-387.

Bacci, M. 2014. *The Many Faces of Christ Portraying the Holy in the East and West, 300-1300.* London: Reaktion.

Betancourt, R. 2018. *Sight, Touch and Imagination in Byzantium.* Cambridge: Cambridge University Press.

Bober, P. P., and Rubinstein, R. 2010. *Renaissance Artists and Antique Sculpture: A Handbook of Sources* (2nd edition). London: Brepols.

Brajović, S., and J. Erdeljan, 2015. 'Praying with the Senses: Examples of Icon Devotion and the Sensory Experience in Medieval and Early Modern Balkans', *ЗОГРАФ* 39: 57-63.

Brubaker, L. 1998. 'Icons before Iconoclasm?', *Morfologie sociali e culturali in europa fra tarda antichità e alto medioevo*, Settimane di Studio del Centro Italiano di Studi sull'Alto Medioevo 45: 1215-1254.

Brubaker, L. 2006. 'In the Beginning Was the Word: Art and Orthodoxy at the Councils of Trullo (692) and Nicaea II (787)' in A. Louth and A. Casiday (eds), *Byzantine Orthodoxies*. Aldershot: Ashgate. pp. 95–101.

Brubaker, L., and Haldon, J. 2011. *Byzantium in the Iconoclast Era c. 680–850: A History*. Cambridge: Cambridge University Press.

Cameron, A. 1984. 'The History of the Image of Edessa: The Telling of a Story' in C. Mango and O. Pritsak (eds), *Okeanos: Essays Presented to Ihor Sevcenko on His Sixtieth Birthday by His Colleagues and Students*. Cambridge, MA: Harvard Research Institute. pp. 80–94.

Caseau, B. 2016. 'Experiencing the Sacred' in Nesbitt and Jackson (2016: 59–77).

Cormack, R., and Vassilaki, M. (eds) 2008. *Byzantium 330-1453*. London: Royal Academy of Arts.

Cross, S. H. 1930. *The Russian Primary Chronicle*. Cambridge, MA: Harvard University Press.

Cross, S. H., and Sherbowitz-Wetzor, O. (eds and transl.) 1953. *Russian Primary Chronicle: Laurentian Text*. Cambridge, MA: Medieval Academy of America.

Cunningham, M. 2014: 'The Impact of ps-Dionysius the Aeropagite on Byzantine Theologians of the Eighth Century: the Concept of "Image"' in J. A. Mihoc and L. Aldea (eds), *A Celebration of Living Theology: A Festschrift in Honour of Andrew Louth*. London: Bloomsbury. pp. 41–58.

Ćurčić, S. Ć., and Hadjitryphonos, E. (eds) 2010. *Architecture as Icon: Perception and Representation of Architecture in Byzantine Art*. New Haven: Yale University Press.

Cutler, A. 1995. 'From Loot to Scholarship: Changing Modes in the Italian Response to Byzantine Artifacts, ca. 1200–1750,' *Dumbarton Oaks Papers* 49: 237–267. https://doi.org/10.2307/1291714

De Vere, G. du C. (ed. and transl.) 1996. *Giorgio Vasari: Lives of the Painters, Sculptors and Architects* (2 vols). New York: Everyman's Library.

Demus, O. 1948. *Byzantine Mosaic Decoration: Aspects of Monumental Art in Byzantium*. London: Paul, Trench, Trubner.

Eastmond, A. 2013. *The Glory of Byzantium and Early Christendom*. London: Phaidon.

Evans, H. C. 2004. *Byzantium: Faith and Power (1261–1557)*. New Haven: Yale University Press.

Guscin, M. 2009. *The Image of Edessa*. Leiden: Brill.

Hadjinicolaou, N. 2008. 'La defensa del arte bizantino por El Greco: notas sobre una paradoja,' *Archivo Español de Arte* 323: 217–232. Online English translation (including photograph):
http://www.sciencedaily.com/releases/2008/12/081218132252.htm (accessed 22 June 2017).

Hahn, C., and Klein, H.A. (eds) 2015. *Saints and Sacred Matter: The Cult of Relics in Byzantium and Beyond*. Cambridge, MA: Harvard University Press.

James, L. 2011. '"Seeing is Believing, but Feeling's the Truth": Touch and the Meaning of Byzantine Art' in A. Lymberopoulou (ed.), *Images of the Byzantine World. Visions, Messages and Meanings: Studies Presented to Leslie Brubaker*. Farnham: Ashgate. pp. 1–14.

James, L. 2016. 'Things: Art and Experience in Byzantium' in Nesbitt and Jackson (2016: 17–33).

James, M. R. 1924. *The Apocryphal New Testament being the Apocryphal Gospels, Acts, Epistles, and Apocalypses*. Oxford: Clarendon Press.

Kazhdan, A. P. (ed.) 1991. *The Oxford Dictionary of Byzantium* (3 vols). Oxford: Oxford University Press.

Kuryluk, E. 1991. *Veronica and Her Cloth: History, Symbolism and Structure of a 'True' Image*. Oxford: Blackwell.

Louth, A. 2016: 'Experiencing the Liturgy in Byzantium' in Nesbitt and Jackson (2016: 79–88).

Lymberopoulou, A. 2006. *The Church of the Archangel Michael at Kavalariana: Art and Society on Fourteenth-Century Venetian-Dominated Crete*. London: Pindar Press.

Lymberopoulou, A. 2007. 'Audiences and Markets for Cretan Icons' in K. W. Woods, C. M. Richardson and A. Lymberopoulou (eds), *Viewing Renaissance Art*. New Haven: Yale University Press. pp. 171–206.

Lymberopoulou, A., Harrison, L., and Ambers, J. 2011. 'The *Noli Me Tangere* Icon at the British Museum: Vision, Message and Reality' in A. Lymberopoulou (ed.), *Images of the Byzantine World. Visions, Messages and Meanings: Studies Presented to Leslie Brubaker*. Farnham: Ashgate. pp. 185–214.

Maguire, H. 1996. *Icons of their Bodies: Saints and their Images in Byzantium*. Princeton: Princeton University Press.

Mango, C. 1986. *The Art of the Byzantine Empire 312–1453: Sources and Documents*. Toronto: University of Toronto Press.

Mouriki, D. 1970–1972. 'The Theme of the "Spinario" in Byzantine Art', Δελτίον της Χριστιανικής Αρχαιολογικής Εταιρείας ser. 4, 6: 53–66.

Nelson, R. S. 2007a. 'Image and Inscription: Please for Salvation in Spaces of Devotion' in L. James (ed.), *Art and Text in Byzantine Culture*. Cambridge: Cambridge University Press. pp. 100–119.

Nelson, R. S., 2007b. *Later Byzantine Painting: Art, Agency, and Appreciation*. Aldershot: Ashgate.

Nesbitt, C., and Jackson, M. 2016. *Experiencing Byzantium. Papers from the 44th Spring Symposium of Byzantine Studies, Newcastle and Durham, April 2011*. London: Routledge.

Nickell, J. 2007. *Relics of the Christ*. Lexington: The University Press of Kentucky.

Osborne, J, 2003. 'Images of the Mother of God in Early Medieval Rome' in A. Eastmond and L. James (eds), *Icon and the Word: The Power of Images in Byzantium, Studies Presented to Robin Cormack*. Aldershot: Ashgate. pp. 135–156.

Peers, G. 2012. 'Mask, Marriage and the Byzantine Mandylion: Classical Inversions in tenth-century *Narratio de Translatione Constantinopolim Imaginis Edessenae*', Σύμμεικτα Зборник радова поводом четрдесет година Института за историју уметности Филозофског факултета Универзитета у Београду [*Collection of Papers Dedicated to the 40th Anniversary of the Institute for Art History, Faculty of Philosophy, University of Belgrade*]. Belgrade: Faculty of Philosophy, University of Belgrade. pp. 45–54.

Pentcheva, B. V. 2010. *The Sensual Icon: Space Ritual and the Senses in Byzantium*. Philadelphia: The Pennsylvania State University Press.

Pentcheva, B. V. 2011. 'Hagia Sophia and Multisensory Aesthetics', *Gesta* 50.2: 93–111. https://doi.org/10.2307/41550552

Petsopoulos, Y. (ed.) 2016. *Art from the Christian East 400–1500 AD*. London: AXIA.

Richardson, C. M., Woods, K. W., and Franklin, M. W. (eds) 2007. *Renaissance Art Reconsidered an Anthology of the Sources.* Oxford: Blackwell.

Spanke, D. 2000. *Das Mandylion. Ikonographie, Legenden und Bildtheorie der 'Nicht-von-Menschenhand-gamachten Christusbilder'.* Recklinghausen: Museen der Stadt Recklinghausen.

Spatharakis, I. 2010. *Byzantine Wall Painting of Crete, Vol. II: Mylopotamos Province.* Leiden: Alexandros Press.

Tischendorf, C. (ed.) 1959 [1853]. Ευαγγέλια Απόκρυφα. Επί τη Βάσει Ελληνικών και Λατινικών Κωδίκων [*Gospels Archaic: On the Basis of Greek and Latin Codes*]. Athens.

Wolf, G., Dufour Bozzo, C., and Calderoni Masetti, A. R. (eds) 2004. *Mandylion Intorno al Sacro Volto da Bisanzio a Genova.* Milan and Genoa: Skira.

Woods, K. W. 2013. 'Byzantine Icons in the Netherlands, Bohemia and Spain during the Fourteenth and Fifteenth Centuries' in A. Lymberopoulou and R. Duits (eds), *Byzantine Art and Renaissance Europe.* Farnham: Ashgate. pp. 135–155.

Angeliki Lymberopoulou is Senior Lecturer in Byzantine art and culture at The Open University, UK. She is primarily interested in cross-cultural interaction between Byzantine East and Latin West. Her research focuses primarily on the social and religious concerns of artists and patrons as reflected in the artistic production of Crete under Venetian domination (1211–1669) and to what extent this production is indicative of and directly related to the trading industry in the island during this period.

Chapter 6

'Seeing' My Beloved:
Darśan and the Sikhi Perspective

OPINDERJIT KAUR TAKHAR

ਕਾਗਾ ਕਰੰਗ ਢੰਢੋਲਿਆ ਸਗਲਾ ਖਾਇਆ ਮਾਸੁ ॥
ਏ ਦੁਇ ਨੈਨਾ ਮਤਿ ਛੁਹਉ ਪਿਰ ਦੇਖਨ ਕੀ ਆਸ ॥੯॥[1]

The crows have searched my skeleton, and eaten all my flesh.
But please do not touch these eyes; I hope to see my Beloved.
— Guru Granth Sahib (GGS), Ang/page 1382

Sikhi, by which I refer to the teachings primarily contained in the Guru Granth Sahib (GGS), are replete with references to the eyes and for a longing to 'see' the Divine, often referred to as the Groom and the Beloved. The term generally used for this 'vision' in Indian philosophy is *darśan*, derived from a verb root *dr̥ś*, 'to see', therefore implying a vision of the Divine, and also a vision of Reality. My discussion will focus on the concept of *darśan* from a Sikh perspective. One is inevitably, at this point, faced with the rather large task of providing a definition of Sikh identity which satisfactorily encompasses the diversity within the Sikh Panth (the global community of Sikhs), in terms of both belief and practice. In common to all faiths, Sikh practices too tend to be defined as either mainstream or sectarian. In keeping with current trends around 'lived religion', I will address the diversity in terms of the practical application of *darśan* amongst the wider Sikh community, particularly so in the section dealing with Sants and Babas. A

---

1 References in the Gurmukhi font have been accessed from the SriGranth Online Resource developed by Punjabi University Patiala. Accessible at: www.srigranth.org (accessed 13 June 2017).

detailed insight into perspectives on Sikh identity can be found in Takhar (2005) and Singh and Barrier (1999). There is an abundance of published work available which focuses on the concept of *darśan* within the Hindu way of life as both an emphasis on 'seeing and being seen' by the Divine through *murtis*, images representing the various forms of the Ultimate Brahman, as well as the concept of *darśan* as a 'vision' of Reality which is unpacked through the Six Philosophical Schools of Indian Thought, the *Darśanas* (Eck 1998; Flood 1996; Fowler 2016). Indeed, in discussing *darśan*, it has often been stated that '[T]he premise in the Hindu religion is that the deity inhabits the statue' (Rutherford 2000: 145). With its emphasis on the transcendent Ultimate Reality, there is no scope in Sikh teachings and philosophy for 'seeing' the Divine through *murtis*; quite simply, there are no images of the Divine according to Sikh teachings. Essentially, Sikhi refers to the Divine as gender-free. Nevertheless, in a metaphorical sense, the reference to the Divine as the Groom and to humanity as a whole as the bride is gendered. So, how is the concept of *darśan* to be understood from the Sikh perspective?

I will attempt, in what follows, to make sense of the importance of the sense of sight, of 'seeing', in Sikh teachings as embodied in the eternal Guru for the majority of Sikhs – the Guru Granth Sahib. My discussion will also explore the lived aspect of *darśan* for Sikhs in contemporary society. Any building which houses the Guru Granth Sahib becomes a gurdwara, the Sikh place of worship, literally translated as the 'door/gateway to the Guru'. Unarguably, gurdwaras are central to Sikh communities, wherever in the world they have settled. The dedication with which gurdwaras are built is indicative of the importance of physically seeing the Guru Granth Sahib, that is having its *darśan*, since it is meditation and contemplation of the teachings which enable the experiential and numinous 'seeing' of the Divine. The manner in which the Guru Granth Sahib is treated as the eternal *living* Guru is notable (see Cole and Sambhi 1995: 44–57) in order to understand what Sikhs actually *do* in their efforts to have *darśan* of the Divine (see Figure 6.1). The *sangat* or the congregation holds particular importance in Sikh collective worship since this is the environment in which one can be guided by highly respected, spiritual beings. This does not mean, however, that Sikhs are discouraged from quiet individual meditation. *Nam Japna*, meditation on the Name of the Divine is one of the key principles of the Sikh faith. The Guru Granth Sahib uses many Names to refer to the Divine; in popular contemporary practice the Divine is often referred to as *Waheguru*, a name used in the Guru Granth Sahib.

Darśan *and the Sikhi Perspective* 133

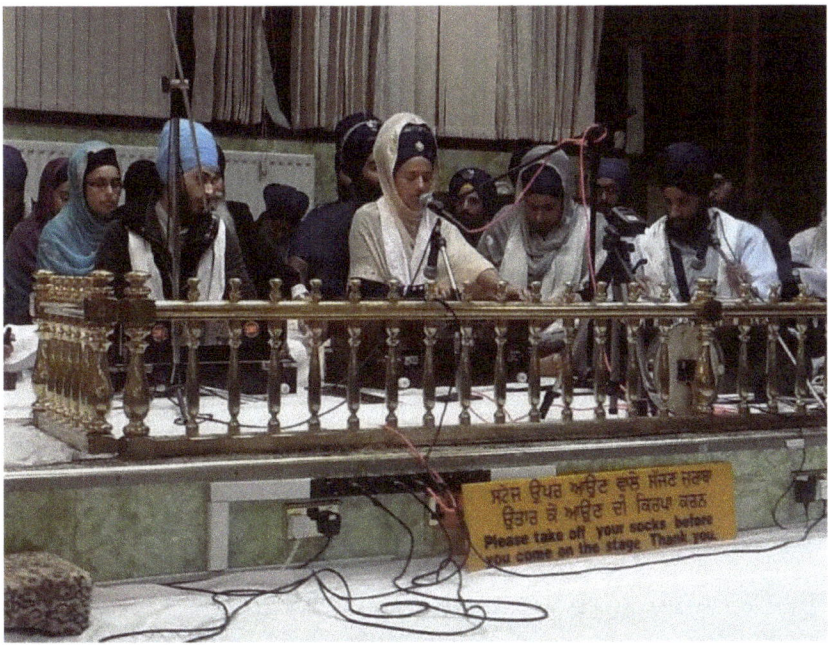

Figure 6.1 *Kirtan* in a gurdwara in the UK. Photograph by Sukhbir Kaur.

Traditional Indian music, using traditional Indian instruments (particularly the harmonium and tabla) is a fundamental aspect of what Sikhs *do*. Here, the sense of hearing is paramount in the singing of *kirtan*, teachings from the Guru Granth Sahib, and occasionally the Dasam Granth (Figure 6.1). It is important to note that the teachings of the Guru Granth Sahib are written in accordance to *ragas*, musical notes, and are therefore intended to be sung (see Bhogal 2011; Cassio 2012). The role of the *ragi*, one who has taken training in the playing of the harmonium and tabla, therefore is essential in communal worship. The sense of smell, like that in the Greek Orthodox Church (see Lymberopoulou in this volume) is also enhanced by the burning of incense in most gurdwaras. Accompanying this is the smell of food which wafts into the main worship hall from the kitchen where *langar* is prepared and served all day long. It is an expectation that all who visit the gurdwara, Sikh and non-Sikh, should partake of the *langar* (the vegetarian meal, free to all visitors and worshippers). Gurdwara attendees are also expected to take *karah prasad*, a sweet and warm semolina and butter blessing which emphasises the concept of equality. Sikhs and non-Sikhs attending the gurdwara, thus, both practically and symbolically,

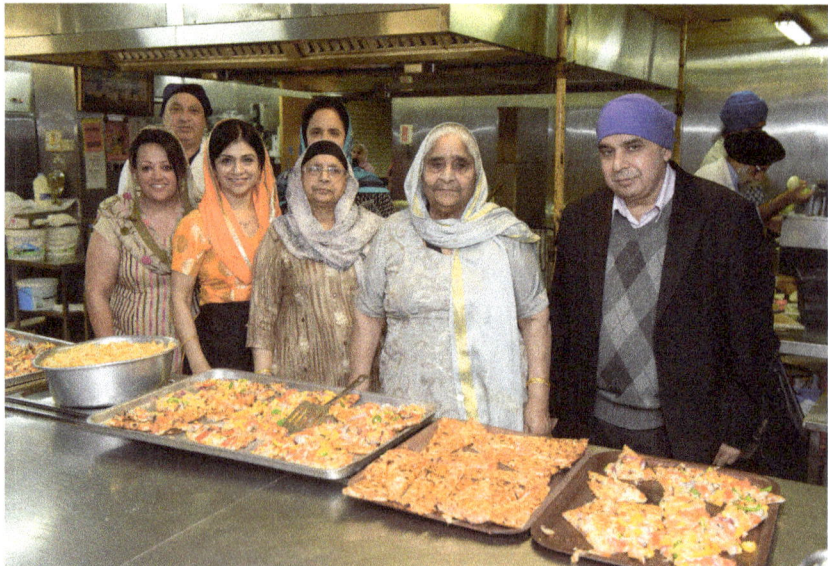

Figure 6.2 Pizza *langar* at Guru Nanak Gurdwara, Wolverhampton. Photograph by Opinderjit Kaur Takhar.

enforce the concept of equality by their actions in partaking of the *karah prasad* and the *langar*. The sense of taste is therefore also used in communal worship. Indeed, it is not unusual for gurdwaras to prepare vegetarian pizza and pasta alongside chips for the *langar* in their efforts to attract the younger generation (figure 6.2).

'SEEING' IS 'KNOWING'?

Core to the teachings of Sikhi is the concept that ultimate release from the cycle of transmigration is the responsibility of the Divine, Ultimate Reality rather than the individual. The term very often used in the Guru Granth Sahib for what roughly translates as 'Grace' is *Nadar* (which has strong connotations of the term *nazar* which means 'sight' or 'vision'). One must remember however, that there are no images of the Divine according to Sikhi, so what exactly does a 'vision' entail according to the hermeneutics of the Guru Granth Sahib?

Time and time again, the teachings of the Guru Granth Sahib allude to the bestowing of *Nadar* as the opportunity to transcend one's consciousness from being *manmukh* (worldly/self-orientated) to *gurmukh* (attuned to the Divine). To become *gurmukh* is the concept of an awakened mind; according to Sikhi, a *gurmukh* is one who has 'seen' the formless Divine, one who has 'heard' the *anahad sabad* (the unstruck melody) which suggests a heightening of the senses, an awakening of the *man/buddhi*. Importantly, in Indian philosophy overall, the term *man* has a much wider connotation than simply the 'mind': the word lacks a satisfactory translation in English, and can also be associated with the heart, which is further allied with feelings and emotions (McLeod 1996). In verbal discourses of the Guru Granth Sahib the term *buddhi* is also often used for both the mind and the conscience. Sikh practice is replete with the singing of the hymns of the Guru Granth Sahib, together with the hearing of *kirtan*, as a practical means towards the calming the *man*. The performance of *kirtan* 'is an art of spiritual communication' with the Divine (Singh 2014: 397). Guru Arjan Dev clearly links *darśan* with an awakening of the *man*:

ਮੇਰਾ ਮਨੁ ਲੋਚੈ ਗੁਰ ਦਰਸਨ ਤਾਈ ॥
My man *longs for the Blessed Vision of the Guru's* darśan.

(GGS, Ang 96)

ਹਰਿ ਦਰਸਨ ਕਉ ਮਨੁ ਲੋਚਦਾ ਨਾਨਕ ਪਿਆਸ ਮਨਾ ॥
My man *yearns for* darśan *of the Divine, Nanak, my mind is thirsty.*

(GGS, Ang 133)

Therefore, 'seeing' according to the Guru Granth Sahib, is a realisation, a mystical experience of the acceptance of the immanence of the Divine within each and every human being. Nikky-Guninder Kaur Singh eloquently equates 'seeing' as realisation of the immanent Divine; for her

> ... *dekhai* or eyesight is, metaphysically speaking, identical with the category of *sujhai* – realization or discovery; literally, being endowed with insight into phenomena as they intrinsically are. Senses and rationality are not pitted against each other; on the contrary, they include each other. (1993: 21)

The emphasis here is upon 'love', a personal relationship with the transcendent Divine through *bhakti* to a gender-free, formless Ultimate Divine, which must be experienced and realised in order to awaken the conscience into the ideal state of a *gurmukh*. *Nadar*, with its synonym *darśan*, is conceived of as a gift to humanity, an opportunity to experience *sahaj*, the mystical union with the Divine through *Nam Simran* which is contemplation and meditation on the Name. An analysis of the teachings of the Guru

Granth Sahib indicates that *sahaj* is the resulting mystical experience of receiving *darśan* (Takhar 2005: 43–45), which in turn suggests that *sahaj* and *darśan* are coterminous. *Darśan* is thus the realisation of the Truth, an absence of which brings sadness and suffering. The pursuit to end such suffering became a central concern for Guru Nanak (McLeod 1996: 162). The concept of *chardi kala* amongst Sikhs refers to 'high spirits/overcoming anxiety' and is synonymous with the controlling of the *man*. Sikh spiritual leaders very often prescribe the hearing of *kirtan* as the path towards *chardi kala* and therefore combatting mental illness and depression.

In practice, these teachings are encompassed in the practice of meditation – both on the Name, *Nam Japna*, as well as in the form of *kundalini yoga*. The practice of the latter has become visibly present amongst Sikhs through the efforts of Harbhajan Singh Khalsa, popularly known as Yogi Bhajan. It is through the efforts of Yogi Bhajan in the 1970s onwards in America that the Panth has seen an influx of non-Punjabi Sikhs (Takhar 2005: 158–178). There are numerous gurdwaras across the globe offering classes on *kundalini yoga*. For many Sikhs, the practical aspect of teachings around 'seeing' the Divine is through the mystical experience of Union with the immanent *Waheguru* – an experience derived through such practices as *kundalini yoga* in which the climax of 'seeing the truth' is to open the tenth gate of consciousness. The numinosity and ineffability, to use Rudolf Otto's terms, of 'seeing' the Divine transcends the conscience to its highest point, that of the *dasam duar*, the tenth gate, the highest *chakra* according to Nath yogic terminology, which is also used by Guru Nanak in his teachings. The point is succinctly illustrated by Hew McLeod:

> Ascending to higher and yet higher levels of spiritual perception he [humankind] finally reaches the ultimate, a condition of ineffable union with the Eternal One in which all earthly bonds are dissolved and the cycle of death and rebirth finally brought to an end. (1996: 150–51)

Indeed such teachings form the core of *kundalini yoga* for many Sikhs across the world today. McLeod goes on to state that *sahaj* is 'the ineffable radiance beyond the *dasam duar*' (1996: 225). An ineffable experience can only be understood by those whom have themselves experienced it. Here again we find a connection to the concept of the *anahad sabad*, the 'unstruck melody' which can only be heard by one who has received the *Nadar*, and therefore a recipient of the *darśan* of the Divine, indeed an experience that is referred to in the teachings of Guru Nanak and directly linked to his own mystical union in his vision of the Divine. McLeod is of the opinion that *sahaj* is a 'word which at once carries us back into Nath theory and beyond the Nath tradition into the earlier world of tantric Buddhism'. (1996: 153)

The term *visamad* refers to the feeling of being in awe in the presence of the Divine, unarguably the result of having *darśan* of the Divine through a mystical experience. 'Seeing' therefore is the absorption of the *man*, through *Nam Simran*, into unity with the Divine, in a inseparable relationship based on utmost love that the bride (symbolising humanity) feels at the 'sight' of her Beloved Groom (an allegory for the Divine). The metaphor of a wedding day, in which the bride longs to be united with her Beloved Groom is used on a number of occasions in the Guru Granth Sahib to depict the relationship between humanity and the Divine. The Guru Granth Sahib highlights the ecstatic feelings of the bride when united with her groom; it also illustrates her sorrow and sadness when separated from him. This is a concept that finds expression in the teachings of the Northern Sant tradition and referred to as *viraha/birha*. Hence meditation on the Name of the Beloved is a remedy for the bride's longing to 'see' her groom:

> [T]he practice of *nam simaran* results in experiences which develop progressively as meditation draws the individual nearer and nearer to God, and which find their ultimate perfection in the final absorption of the *man* into Him. The experience of *visamad* is, in this way, both a result of *nam simaran* and a stimulus to more exalted meditation. (McLeod 1996: 219)

In an exploration of the hermeneutics of the Guru Granth Sahib, one finds an inseparable connection between the terms *Hukam* and *Nadar*. *Hukam* is translated as the Will of the Divine, in accordance to which the *atman/jiva*, the eternal self, is granted birth into the human realm, thus bestowed with the golden opportunity to realise the Divine, to have a vision of Ultimate Reality. Indeed, the *gurmukh* is characterised by total submission to the *Hukam* (GGS, Ang 636). According to Gavin Flood, since the root verb for *darśan* is *dr̥ś*, 'to see', the term therefore implies a vision of the world, of Ultimate Reality (1996: 224), and this finds a repeated expression in the teachings of the Guru Granth Sahib. *Darśan* from the Sikhi perspective therefore is not to be within the gaze of the Divine through *puja* to a *murti*, but rather to live in accordance with the *Hukam* through selfless service, *Nam Simran*, and a total submission to Ultimate Reality through *bhakti*. It is thus through *Nadar* that the experience of 'meeting' the Divine through *darśan* is bestowed upon the *gurmukh*. Individual effort is paramount in the bestowal of *Nadar*, *darśan* of the Divine is therefore the fruit of one's selfless actions and *bhakti* through *Nam Simran*:

ਤੇਰੇ ਦਰਸਨ ਕਉ ਬਲਿਹਾਰਣੈ ਤੁਸਿ ਦਿਤਾ ਅੰਮ੍ਰਿਤੁ ਨਾਮੁ

I would sacrifice myself for your darśan, *you have blessed me with the Ambrosial Name of the Divine.*

(GGS, Ang 52)

According to Sikh tradition, teachings, or the 'word' (*bani*) concerning the Ultimate Divine and knowledge relating to Reality were revealed to Guru Nanak during a three-day disappearance when he was taken to the 'court' of the Divine. This marks the beginning of Nanak's Guruship, during which he, accompanied by his two closest companions, Mardana and Bala, imparted that divinely received knowledge and wisdom to his followers. It is this 'seeing' of the totally formless and transcendent Divine by Guru Nanak which marks the genesis of the Sikh Faith, 'a vision which formed the foundations of the Sikh religion' (Kaur Singh 1993: 18). Kaur Singh goes on to compare Guru Nanak's experience with that of Arjuna's cosmic vision of the Divine in the *Bhagavad Gita* (ibid.). Whereas Arjuna's experience is described as the imparting of knowledge of the infinite forms of the Divine, for Guru Nanak *darśan* is the experience of Ultimate knowledge by realising the all-pervading nature of *Akal Purakh*, one of the many names for the Ultimate Divine used in the Guru Granth Sahib. Teachings emphasising the formless nature of the Divine are, therefore, fundamental to Sikh belief. Indeed, the feminine principle in the Sikh vision of the transcendent presents a 'holistic way of imagining and experiencing sacred power that can itself be a mode of [female] empowerment' (ibid.: 5). Mandair further places emphasis upon the *experiential* aspect of Ultimate Reality, as something that is '*experienced* all the time, rather than simply comprehended' (2013: 135). Here again the practical application of such teachings is expressed through the practices of *Nam Japna* and the singing and hearing of *kirtan* for its aesthetic as well as mystical experience of *darśan*.

The concept of the unity of the Divine according to Sikhi is one which sees the world, indeed the universe, and every material aspect of creation as existing within the Ultimate Divine. Hence, the Divine is both personal, and yet also totally transcendent. The Guru Granth Sahib conceptualises the Divine as *nirguna*, which essentially alludes to the Divine as being formless, transcendent and incomprehensible. Nevertheless, one of Sikhi's core principles is that of the importance of *bhakti* as essential in the *man's* longing for *darśan*. In this respect the Divine becomes *saguna*, manifest in creation, so that human beings can experience *sahaj*, union with the immanent Divine. Those who ignore the initial *Nadar*, which is the granting of the human birth, remain on the ignorant level of a *manmukh*, whereas the *gurmukh* is one characterised by the loss of the *haumai*, the ego, and portrays a higher level of consciousness in their daily conduct through the experience of the *darśan* of *Waheguru*:

ਮੇਰੀ ਅਹੰ ਜਾਇ ਦਰਸਨ ਪਾਵਤ ਹੇ ॥

My ego is gone; I have obtained the Blessed Vision of darśan.

(GGS, Ang 830)

In this respect, *darśan* according to Sikhi, is both 'seeing' as well as 'being seen' by the Divine (Beckerlegge 2001). Guru Arjan clearly makes the point that 'seeing' is indeed the realisation of the immanent Divine:

ਸੇ ਨੇਤ੍ਰ ਪਰਵਾਣੁ ਜਿਨੀ ਦਰਸਨੁ ਪੇਖਾ ॥

Those eyes which behold darśan *are approved and accepted.*

(GGS, Ang 103)

Nadar, which is also expressed as *nazar*, 'vision', is thus expressed as 'Grace', a gift from the Divine; *Nadar* is essentially to 'be seen' by the Divine (GGS, Ang 465). 'Seeing' is used metaphorically as 'knowing'; both terms are fundamentally linked to one another. The Sanskrit translation of the term *darśana*, as noted above, alludes to both the Six Schools of Indian Philosophy (knowledge), as well as a vision of the Divine (sight). Furthermore, 'the Sanskrit root *vid*, meaning "to know", is etymologically related to the Latin *videre* = to see, and to the Greek *oida* = to know ...' (Kaur Singh 1993: 20).

For Guru Ram Das, good fortune, which we may interpret as the bestowal of *Nadar*, is inextricably linked to good deeds; those individuals who fail to recognise the *Hukam* are indeed unfortunate, since *darśan* is a vision of Reality for the fortunate to perceive the Truth:

ਬਿਨੁ ਭਾਗਾ ਦਰਸਨੁ ਨਾ ਥੀਐ ਭਾਗਹੀਣ ਬਹਿ ਰੋਇ ॥

Darśan *is unattainable without good fortune, the unfortunate sit and cry.*

(GGS, Ang 41)

This would imply that the repudiation of *darśan* brings misery since the *manmukh* remains attached to the temporary lures of the physical world; the term used for this attachment in the Guru Granth Sahib is *maya*. *Maya* here is not the world-rejecting concept found in the monism of *advaita*; rather Sikhi teaches that the created world is very much real – it is the *karam bhumi*, the action ground, in which the individual transcends, through effort, the conscience to that of the level of the *gurmukh*, at which *darśan* results in the experiencing and realising of the formless Divine:

ਨੇਤ੍ਰ ਪੁਨੀਤ ਪੇਖਤ ਹੀ ਦਰਸ ॥
My eyes are purified, beholding the Blessed Vision of darśan.

(GGS, Ang 201)

Darśan in popular Sikh practice also refers to the physical act of bowing down, in respect, to the Guru Granth Sahib. This is usually carried out in the gurdwara, where the burning of incense activates the mind in sacred space. In this respect, *darśan* is indeed the vision (knowledge) of the Divine, as encapsulated in the revealed *bani* of the Gurus and the Hindu and Muslim Bhagats whose *bani* is contained in the eternal Guru of the Sikhs. It is useful to repeat here that the term gurdwara translates as the 'door to the Guru', that is to the eternal Guru installed within the throne-like structure of the *palki*. A gurdwara is not 'the house of God'. The very use of the term 'God' is problematic in the Sikh context due to its masculine connotations which contradict the gender-free and utterly formless Divine according to the Sikhi perspective.

Returning to the *darśan* of the Guru Granth Sahib, the implications of its online availability deserve a mention. Sikhs go to great lengths to preserve the sanctity of the eternal Guru such as placing it at a higher level, covering it in special cloths (*rumalas*) and other practical measures with underlying symbolic significance which emphasise its status of royalty and hence utmost importance. A tremendous level of care and respect is undertaken by Sikhs to avoid any *beadbi*, disrespect, towards the eternal Guru. But how does this operate in cyberspace? How does one ensure that there is no *beadbi* towards the online Guru? Scheifinger (2008) explores the implications of *darśan* online for Hindus and acknowledges some interesting issues associated with online authority in the Hindu world; however, this is often overlooked in relation to online versions of the Guru Granth Sahib.

THE INSEPARABLE RELATIONSHIP BETWEEN *BHAKTI* AND *DARŚAN*

The human predicament is the *atman*'s (the eternal self/soul's) entrapment in *samsara*, the cycle of continuous death and rebirth. Such transmigration of the eternal self is the result of attachment to worldly pleasures, as characterized by the predominance of the *haumai*, the ego. As remarked earlier, birth into the human realm is, according to the Guru Granth Sahib, the golden opportunity through which the Divine can be realised through *darśan* (GGS, Ang 176), which is synonymous with *Nadar*, the gift of 'vision'. It is emphasised however, that the human birth is regarded as the highest of all births in Sikhism. It is the human birth alone, through which individual effort is of paramount importance towards *mukti*, the atman's release from the cycle of *samsara*. Since the *haumai* is the obstacle in Divine realisation, it must be overcome through a personal and loving relationship with the Divine through *bhakti*. Contemplation on the Name of the Divine, which has become the core foundation of *Nam Simran* in Sikhi, is a distinguishing pillar of Sikh thought. Hence the path, the *marga*, of *bhakti* is placed on a pedestal in Sikh philosophy. However, the final release from *samsara* is dependent wholly upon the bestowal of *Nadar*, individual efforts alone cannot guarantee *mukti*. The *manmukh* remains alienated from the Divine and chooses not to respond to the bestowal of *darśan/Nadar*, and hence remains bound to the cycle of *samsara*.

The path to God involves primarily meditation upon the Name of God, that is *Nam Simran*. The *gurmukh* who meditates upon the *Nam* (Name) stands in opposition to the five vices of *kam* (lust), *krodh* (anger), *lobh* (greed), *moh* (attachment) and *ahankar* (pride). Meditation on the Name enables the *gurmukh* to become detached from the *samsaric* hold of worldly attachments. The path towards *mukti* can also be found through *Sabad*, listening to the words of the Guru Granth Sahib. The concept of *Sabad* was incorporated into Guru Nanak's theology from the Northern Sant tradition, to describe the mystical 'sound' experienced at the climax of the *hatha-yoga* technique (McLeod and Schomer 1987: 229–250).

What then is the ultimate deciding factor in whether a vision of the Divine is granted? Is it human effort or Divine Grace? Surely, in order for the human birth to be regarded as the golden opportunity to 'see' the Divine, effort on part of the individual is paramount? This dilemma is examined in the context of what is known as the *panj khand*. This is the transition from the *manmukh* to the *gurmukh* via five stages or 'realms'. The *panj khand* concept unites both concepts of individual effort and Divine 'Grace' in 'seeing' and thus realising the Divine through each evolutionary stage in elevating the conscience to the higher level. The first stage is that of *Dharam khand*, an understanding of the law of cause and effect in the universe both physically and morally. This stage is where the Divine has bestowed *Nadar* on the *atman* to be reborn into the human realm. The next *khand* is that of *Gian*, translated as the realm of knowledge (*gian* is synonymous with the term *jnana* in a dualistic understanding of Reality) in the sense that it widens an individual's spiritual consciousness. It is in this realm that one's *haumai* is overcome as a result of acknowledging the *Hukam*. The third stage in the progression of elevated consciousness is that of *Saram khand* – the realm of effort. This inevitably is the stage of selfless actions and utmost devotion to the Divine as a result of the vision of the Divine through *darśan*. The next evolutionary stage is that of *Karam khand*, the realm of Ultimate *Nadar*. The ultimate goal of Sikhi is to enter the final and fifth realm of Truth, *Sach khand*. This is the realm of the *jivanmukt*, the one whose *atman* has united with the Divine. Importantly, this five-stage transition is based on the concept of dualism, where the Divine is always over and above all that has been created.

DARŚAN OF SANTS AND BABAS

The term Sant, used interchangeably with Baba in a Punjabi context, refers to a person of spiritual piety, and bears similarity to the concept and role of a Saint in popular usage. The role of the Sant and/or Baba is becoming increasingly important in contemporary Sikh practice in relation to the concept of *darśan*. Living Sants and Babas are becoming the channels through which many Sikhs perceive *darśan* very much in the context of *seeing and being seen* (Eck 1998: 3). Followers of such Sants and Babas flock in their masses to have *darśan*, 'to see' these perceived personifications of elevated conscience, very often conceived of as possessing divinity themselves in the eyes of their followers. It would thus not be incorrect to label many of these followers as the devotees of such individuals whom are believed to have powers to bestow *darśan* on their followers (Cox and Robinson 2006). Although Sikhi is generally cautious about such elevated individuals, many Sants and Babas in the Sikh context have become rather renowned for a 'back to Sikhi' approach, as Tatla highlights:

> Among the factors which have sustained the religious and cultural orientation of Sikhs in Britain, the role of the visiting Sants is of crucial importance. Sants have shaped the lives of many of their Sikh disciples directly, inspiring others to uphold the religious ideals, and have contributed in several ways to the community's causes and institutions (1992: 349).

Diversity amongst the Sikhs in relation to Sant-orientated groups have been discussed in Takhar (2005). Of particular importance here are the Namdharis and the followers of the Sants of the Nishkam Sewak Jatha. The former are often regarded as heretics by the Panth (global Sikh community) since they explicitly refer to their leaders as Gurus, in continuation of the line of Sikh human Gurus, thus rejecting the fundamental Sikh belief in the Guru Granth Sahib as the eternal Guru of the Sikhs, as proclaimed by Guru Gobind Singh in 1708 CE. Takhar (2005: 59–88) provides a detailed discussion of the Namdhari rejection of the Adi Granth[2] as the eternal Guru of the Sikhs. Namdharis do not place the Adi Granth in the *palki*, and *darśan* in their places of worship, referred to as *bhawans*, revolves around a photograph of the present living Guru in his physical absence. The Namdhari Guru is believed to possess divine powers to bestow *darśan* on his followers. His visit to Britain for example, is a time for British Namdharis to assemble in a mass in order to have 'sight' of him and thus receive his blessing (Takhar 2014: 354–356).

The leaders of the Nishkam Sewak Jatha are referred to as Sants and Babas rather than Gurus. In this respect the Nishkam Sewak Jatha and its followers are readily accepted as Sikhs within the Panth at large, due to the fact that they revere the Guru Granth Sahib as the eternal Guru and place great emphasis on becoming initiated into the Khalsa fold. However, the position of their Sants and Babas, amongst followers, is an indication of their belief that *darśan* of the present living Baba, Mohinder Singh, is akin to being bestowed with Divine blessings (see Takhar 2005: 38–58).

Both Baba Mohinder Singh, as well as the Namdhari Guru, Udhay Singh, are able to physically see and touch their followers, and they are believed to be, in the eyes of their followers, direct pathways to the Divine. In this respect, the senses of touch and sight both become relevant in the bestowal of *darśan* in the contemporary sense of living Gurus, Sants and Babas (Eck 1998: 9). Cox and Robinson's (2006) detailed study of the Sachkand Nanak Dham Sants, as well as Nesbitt's research on the Nanaksar Sants (1985) also observe such veneration of living spiritual leaders by their devotees and followers. Juergensmeyer, through his work on the Radhasoami Sants, the followers/adherents of whom float on the fuzzy boundaries between Punjabi Hindu and Sikh identity,[3] succinctly states that:

---

2 The term Adi Granth was used for the Sikh scripture when it was compiled by the fifth Guru Arjan in 1603–1604. In 1708, according to popular Sikh belief, it became the eternal Guru for the Sikhs, hence the term Guru Granth Sahib was used. Because the Namdharis deny this belief, they do not acknowledge the Adi Granth as the eternal Guru.

3 The fuzzy boundaries between Hindu, Sufi and Sikh Identity are particularly relevant to the Sindhi community. See Ramey (2008).

> [a]mong village followers of the movement especially, the sacred sight (*darśan*) of the living Master has powerful, even healing qualities. I have seen mothers rush to hold up their sick children as the automobile of the present Master ... hurries past .... (1987: 342).

The concept of *darśan* thus remains pivotal in many Indian traditions which may not sit neatly within the boundary of either being Hindu or Sikh, a further example of which is the Wolverhampton-based *Ek Niwas* following of Baba Balaknath (see Takhar and Jacobs 2011). LaBrack's observation of the veneration of Sikhs towards living Sants in America, is easily transferable to beliefs amongst Sikhs on a global level. He states:

> [T]he presence of a Sant is in itself edifying and a spiritual boost to the community. The ideas and concepts associated with *darśan* are still very much alive, even among second-generation American-born Punjabi Sikh children .... (1987: 266).

He also makes the point, however, that such veneration is not supported in the teachings of Sikhi (ibid.: 268).

In conclusion, Sikhi – that is the body of teachings primarily from the Guru Granth Sahib – acknowledges that 'seeing' the formless, incomprehensible Divine involves utmost acceptance of the Divine Will, the *Hukam*. A prerequisite to such knowledge is the abandonment of the ego, the *haumai*. With its etymology in the Sanskrit root *dṛś* (to see/vision), *darśan* in its relation to a 'sight and seeing' is the sense that is discussed at length in the Indian religions, particularly Hindu and Sikh, and all those that fall within the blurred boundaries which lie between the two. So how does 'seeing' the divine through a *murti* compare with the seeing of the Divine according to Sikhi? For the latter, there are numerous teachings in the Guru Granth Sahib which imply that *darśan* is the 'experiencing' of the immanence of the Divine, 'seeing' the self in relation to Ultimate Reality, where sight is used as a metaphor for the experience of *sahaj*. The practical steps towards *sahaj* and thus *darśan* of the Divine is through practices such as keeping the company of the *sangat*, the singing and hearing of *kirtan*, and individual as well as communal meditation in the form of *Nam Japna* and physical yoga. Sikh sectarian movements with living Sants, Babas and Gurus, have their own unique practices associated with the concept of *darśan*, the most prominent of which are the seeking of blessings from the revered spiritual leader.

REFERENCES

Beckerlegge, G. 2001. 'Hindu Sacred Images for the Mass Market' in G. Beckerlegge (ed.), *From Sacred Text to Internet*. Milton Keynes: Open University Press.

Bhogal, B. S. 2011. 'The Hermeneutics of Sikh Music (Rag) and Word (Shabad)', *Sikh Formations: Religion, Culture, Theory* 7.3: 211–244.
https://doi.org/10.1080/17448727.2011.640420

Cassio, F. 2012. 'The Music of the Sikh Gurus' Tradition in a Western Context', *Sikh Formations: Religion, Culture, Theory* 7.3: 313–337.
https://doi.org/10.1080/17448727.2011.637360

Cole, W. O., and Sambhi, P.S. 1995. *The Sikhs: Their Religious Beliefs and Practices*. Sussex: Sussex Academic Press.

Cox, L., and Robinson, C. 2006. 'The Living Words of the Living Master: Sants, Sikhs, Sachkhand Nanak Dham and the Academy', *Journal of Contemporary Religion* 21.3: 373–387. https://doi.org/10.1080/13537900600926154

Eck, D. 1998. *Darsan: Seeing the Divine Image in India*. New York: Columbia University Press.

Flood, G. 1996. *An Introduction to Hinduism*. Cambridge: Cambridge University Press.

Fowler, J. 2016. *Hinduism: Beliefs and Practices, Volume 2*. Brighton: Sussex Academic Press.

Juergensmeyer, M. 1987. 'The Radhasoami Revival of the Sant Tradition' in McLeod and Schomer (1987: 329–355).

Kaur Singh, N.-G. 1993. *The Feminine Principle in the Sikh Vision of the Transcendent*. Cambridge: Cambridge University Press.
https://doi.org/10.1017/CBO9780511557415

LaBrack, B. 1987. 'Sants and the Sant Tradition in the Context of Overseas Sikh Communities' in McLeod and Schomer (1987: 265–280).

Mandair, A.-P. 2013. *Sikhism: A Guide for the Perplexed*. London: Bloomsbury.

McLeod, W. H. 1996. *Guru Nanak and the Sikh Religion*. Delhi: Oxford University Press.

McLeod, W. H., and Schomer, K. 1987. *The Sants: Studies in a Devotional Tradition of India*. Delhi: Motilal Banarsidass.

Nesbitt, E. 1985. 'The *Nanaksar* Movement', *Religion* 15: 67–79.
https://doi.org/10.1016/0048-721X(85)90060-0

Ramey, S. W. (2008). *Hindu, Sufi or Sikh: Contested Practices and Identifications of Sindhi Hindus in India and Beyond*. New York: Palgrave Macmillan.

Rutherford, I. 2000. 'Theoria and *Darśan*: Pilgrimage and Vision in Greece and India', *Classical Quarterly* 50.1: 133–146. https://doi.org/10.1093/cq/50.1.133

Scheifinger, H. 2008. 'Hinduism and Cyberspace', *Religion* 38: 233–249.
https://doi.org/10.1016/j.religion.2008.01.008

Singh, G. 2014. 'Sikh Music' in P. Singh and L. Fenech (eds), *The Oxford Handbook of Sikh Studies*. Oxford: Oxford University Press. pp. 397–407.
https://doi.org/10.1093/oxfordhb/9780199699308.001.0001

Singh, P., and Barrier, N. G. 1999. *Sikh Identity: Continuity and Change*. New Delhi: Manohar.

Takhar, O. K. 2005. *Sikh Identity: An Exploration of Groups among Sikhs*. Farnham: Ashgate.

Takhar, O. K. 2014. 'Sikh Sects' in P. Singh and L. Fenech (eds), *The Oxford Handbook of Sikh Studies*. Oxford: Oxford University Press. pp. 350–359.
https://doi.org/10.1093/oxfordhb/9780199699308.013.011

Takhar, O. K., and Jacobs, S. 2011. 'Confusing the Issue: Field Visits as a Strategy for Deconstructing Religious Boundaries', *Discourse: Learning and Teaching in Philosophical and Religious Studies* 10.2: 31–44.
https://doi.org/10.5840/discourse20111027

Tatla, D. S. 1992. 'Nurturing the Faithful: The Role of the Sant among Britain's Sikhs', *Religion* 22: 349–374. https://doi.org/10.1016/0048-721X(92)90044-5

Opinderjit Kaur Takhar is Director of the Centre for Sikh and Panjabi Studies at the University of Wolverhampton, UK, and also Senior Lecturer and Head of Religious Studies there. Takhar's academic research is focused around Sikh, Dalit and Punjab Studies, and she teaches modules on Indian Religions and the Philosophy of Religion. She has written extensively on matters and issues in relation to British Sikhs, caste and gender, and is the author of *Sikh Identity: An Exploration of Groups among Sikhs* (Ashgate, 2005) which is used as a key text on Sikh identity in universities across the world. She is also an Editorial Board Member of the peer-reviewed journal *Sikh Formations: Religion, Culture, Theory*, and is Guest Editor (along with Surinder S. Jodhka and Hugo Gorringe) of the Special Issue on Caste of the *Journal of Contemporary South Asia* (2017).

Section Four

HEARING

Chapter 7

Resounding Mysteries:
Sound and Silence in the Eleusinian Soundscape

GEORGIA PETRIDOU

Sound, like breath, is experienced as a movement of coming and going, inspiration and expiration. If that is so, then we should say of the body, as it sings, hums, whistles or speaks, that it is *ensounded*. It is like setting sail, launching the body into sound like a boat on the waves or, perhaps more appropriately, like a kite in the sky.

– Ingold (2007: 12, emphasis in original)[1]

Tim Ingold's description of the materiality of sound brings to mind lines 154–158 from the *parodos* (i.e. the entry song the chorus would sing) of Aristophanes' *Frogs*, where a breath (*pnoē*) of *aulos*[2] music and the rhythmic clapping of hands is described as the standard acoustic accompaniment of the jubilant bands of the initiates (*memyemenoi*) into the Eleusinian Mysteries:

---

1 I thank Mark Porter for this reference and for discussing with me the concept of soundscape. Special thanks go to the editors of the volume for their kind invitation to take part in the original workshop and their pertinent comments on an earlier draft of this article. I am also indebted to Jörg Rüpke and the Max-Weber Kolleg for a generous research fellowship under the auspices of the DFG and FWF-funded International Research Training Group 'Resonant World Relations in Ancient and Modern Socio-Religious Practices' project (shared between the University of Erfurt, Germany and Karl-Franzens University, Graz, Austria), which allowed me to work on this article.
2 There were different kinds of *aulos*, a wind instrument, which according to West (1992: 84) looked and sounded more like an oboe and less like a flute.

Heracles: There a breath of *aulos* music will surround you and you will see a miraculous light, like here, and myrtle-groves and the happy *thiasoi* of men and women and much clapping of the hands.
Dionysus: Who are these people?
Heracles: The initiates ....

Albeit refracted through the lenses of Athenian comedy, the *parodos*[3] of the *Frogs* gives us a snapshot of the spirited auditory experience the public segment of the Eleusinian Mysteria must have been for those partaking. Yet for centuries Eleusis, situated about fourteen miles to the west of Athens, was far better known for the proverbial silence that shrouded the two levels of initiation into the Mysteries of the Goddesses: the *myesis* (usually translated in Latin as *initio* and in English as 'initiation') and the next stage, the *epopteia*.[4] There is no real contradiction here. Both sound and silence, and the stark antithesis between them, are testaments to the polyvalent acoustic landscape, or soundscape, of Eleusis.[5] However, unlike other mystery cults (e.g. the cult of Cybele and Attis) whose soundscapes have been meticulously investigated (Pavolini 2015), the soundscape of Eleusis has received relatively little attention.[6] This is partly due to an emic emphasis on the visual aspect of the Great Mysteries (*Megala Mysteria*) of Demeter and Kore, and partly because it is precisely the visual facet of the Mysteries that has for decades monopolised scholarly attention (e.g. Petridou 2013). The present study is an attempt to put things right on this front and, simultaneously, to look closely at the relational dynamic of the acoustic aspect of Eleusis as it can be surmised from the epigraphic, literary and iconographical evidence. The ultimate aim of this chapter is to join forces with the editors of the volume in unravelling the sensorial richness

---

3 In the *Frogs*, the chorus consists of initiates into the Eleusnian Mysteries. Some scholars have doubted that the initiatory rites referred to are the Great Mysteria of Eleusis and have instead proposed several other alternatives, such as the Lesser Mysteries at Agrae (Hooker 1960; Guarducci 1982); and Lenaea (Tierney 1934/5). Nonetheless, there are several good arguments against these suggestions. Most of them can be found in Graf (1974: 40–50) and Dover (1993: 62, n.13).
4 On the terms primary sources use to describe the various degrees of initiation, see Mylonas (1961: 239), Dowden (1980) and Simms (1990).
5 More on the concept of 'soundscape' can be found in the Introduction to Emerit et al. (2015).
6 There are a couple of notable exceptions that confirm the rule, such as Athanassakis (1976) and, more recently, Seaford (2013).

and diversity of religious practices by focusing on the sonorous setting of Classical and post-Classical Eleusis as a case study.

The term 'soundscape', as coined by the Canadian composer R. Murray Schafer at the end of the 1960s, refers to the part of the acoustic environment that is perceivable by humans. The concept is not entirely unproblematic. Tim Ingold (2007), for instance, believes the term was initially useful as a rhetorical schema that drew attention to a sensory register that had been thus far neglected, but has since then 'outlived its usefulness'. Ingold's main objection to the use of the concept of soundscape is that sound, just like light, is not the object but the medium of our perception: 'it [sic. sound] is what we hear *in* (emphasis in the original)'.[7] However, I use 'soundscape' here with a distinctly anthropological sense[8] to denote the sonic equivalent of landscape, or else to encompass everything to which the ears of those partaking in the public and the secret segments of the Great Mysteries would have been exposed. Most of my analysis will be focused on the natural components of the soundscape as the cultural components are sadly lost to us. Like landscape, soundscape is both a natural and a cultural construct embracing both the spontaneous and the meticulously composed, the improvised and the carefully directed sonic setting. It encompasses ideologies and practices of producing and listening to sounds that were extremely culture-specific.[9]

After a few general remarks about the sonic richness of the Greek cultic scene in general, and Eleusis in particular, the first section of this chapter attempts to roughly reconstruct the Eleusinian 'soundscape' (the words and the sounds made and heard in the public and private segments of the Eleusinian festival, as well as those others which remained unheard) as participants in the Great Mysteries of the Two Goddesses may have perceived it in the Classical and post-Classical periods. Due to space restrictions, the following sections provide a mere snippet of some of the key sonic settings from both the public segment of the festival (as attested in

---

7 On the close correlation between light and sound as media of perception, see Ingold (2000).
8 As in Samuels et al. (2010: 330).
9 For an excellent discussion of these culture-specific components of modern religious experience, see Byron Dueck's contribution (Chapter 8) in this volume. Dueck discusses drum and gospel singing in the sonic setting of North American Indigenous sacred observance with a focus on the Canadian city of Winnipeg.

primary sources) and the secret segment (as can be surmised largely from literary allusions and scholarly speculation).[10]

The final part of the chapter draws on the concept of synchronic and diachronic resonance (Rosa 2012; 2014; 2016) as well as earlier scholarly work on the significance of silence in Greek religion and philosophy (Kippenberg and Stroumsa 1995; Montiglio 2000) and argues that through the centuries Eleusis came to be identified more closely with the proverbial silence that shrouds the rites that were accessible to the initiates. It was Plato's influential reception of Eleusinian language and imagery that led a huge number of post-Classical authors, especially of the Hadrianic and Antonine eras (e.g. Plutarch, Dio and Aelius Aristides), to identify the truth the initiates acquired in the course of the initiatory rites with the primordial philosophical truth and knowledge (van Nuffelen 2007; 2011).

THE GREEK FESTIVALS AND THEIR SONOROUS CULTURE

When I suggest that audio-based religious experiences in Eleusis is an under-researched scholarly topic, I do not overstate my case. The majority of students of Greek Religion, and I am no exception to this rule, have opted for discussions that focus on the visual aspect of the initiatory rites.[11] This tendency can only partly be explained by the emic emphasis on the visual segment of the Mysteries (Petridou 2013; 2015: ch. 6 on 'ritual viewing'). The ephemeral nature of sound in general, and the rather limited evidence regarding the sonic settings of the Greek festivals in particular, have both had an influence in shaping scholarly tendencies. Nonetheless, the late Martin West (1992: 14) cannot have been far from the truth in thinking that, in the Greek-speaking world, music is 'constantly associated with the idea of celebration'. No greater celebration ever existed than that of establishing close proximity and communication with the divine, and, as I have argued elsewhere (Petridou 2015: ch. 6), mysteries (*orgia, mystēria, teletai*, etc. in the original) did indeed provide their participants with an epiphany,

---

10 More information about what the individual days of celebration involved in terms of *dromena* (things done), *dykneimena* (things shown) and *legomena* (things said) can be found in Mylonas (1961: ch. IX); Burkert (1983: 248–299; 1987: ch. 4); Bowden (2010: ch. 1); Bremmer (2014: ch. 1); and Cosmopoulos (2003; 2015: 22–23).
11 A notable exception to this rule is Seaford (2013). See the discussion in the last section of this chapter.

i.e. a close encounter with the divine in all sorts of different forms.[12] Although we do not possess sound recordings and musical scores for these festivals, we have solid epigraphic, literary and iconographical evidence about musical instruments, singing, dancing, clapping of the hands, raising loud voices and cries (human and animal alike) all being conspicuously present in Greek religious festivals (Calame 2001; Kubatzki 2016).

At the heart of the majority of these festivals were (a) a joyous procession (quite often a chariot procession) transporting the visual symbol of the presence of the deity,[13] and (b) sacrifice(s) performed in honour of the deity, and often the subsequent communal ritual dining. The phrase 'procession and sacrifice' (*pompē kai thysia*) becomes almost formulaic in the epigraphic evidence.[14] The procession, with the visual symbol of the divine parading through the streets of a village or a city and thus rendering the whole community co-witnesses of the deity's arrival or departure and participants in the festive occasion, may precede or follow the sacrifice(s) offered to the deity (Graf 1996). Neither the sacrificial procession nor the sacrificial feast could be conceived of as taking place in a sonic void. They were all hugely popular, densely populated, and therefore rather boisterous affairs.

ELEUSINIAN SOUNDSCAPE: THE PUBLIC SEGMENT

Participation in the Eleusinian Great Mysteries in the Attic month of Boedromion (the third month of the Attic calendar corresponding roughly to our September/October) could not have been very different from participation in other festivals in terms of structural organisation, distribution

---

12   Cf. Burkert (1987: 90): 'In religious terms, mysteries provide an immediate encounter with the divine'; and Graf (2003: 255): 'But to prepare for and be allowed direct contact with a divinity is a function of most mystery cults'. See also Bowden (2010: 213), who singles out the establishing of a closer relationship with the divine as one of the major aims of initiation rites, along with gaining a new status.

13   By visual symbol of the presence of the deity I mean any visual representation – from the god's figural statue to his or her aniconic representation – that within a specific cultural and festive context could be interpreted as denoting divine presence. On aniconism, see Gaifmann (2012).

14   The term *thysia* can denote both 'sacrifice' and 'festival'. Compare here Plato's *Timaeus* 26e, where *thysia* describes the festival of Panathenaea. On sacrifice and music, see Ekroth (2002; 2007; 2008); Naiden (2013); and the essays in Hitch and Rutherford (2013).

of human, animal and material resources, and more importantly, sonorous culture. Despite scholarly interest being monopolised by what the initiated saw, participation in the Eleusinian initiatory rites was also, from start to finish, a high-octane auditory affair.

On the fifteenth day of Boedromion, in the Poikile Stoa of Athens, the great priest of Eleusis, the Hierophant, read the proclamation (*prohhēsis*), an event that marked the beginning of the festival (*teletē*). 'Everyone who has clean hands and intelligible (Greek) speech', 'he who is pure from all pollution and whose soul is conscious of no evil and who has lived well and justly', the proclamation specified, could proceed with the initiation; the rest of the people should abstain (Origen's *Contra Celsum* 3.59; Libanius' *Declamations* 13.19, 52; Julian, *Orations* 7.25; with Dickie 2004). The next day was marked by lustrations and purifications in the sea. The famous cry of 'To the sea, initiands!' (*Halade Mystae*) became synonymous with the Eleusinian rites. One can only imagine the deafening cries of the suckling pig, which was purified and subsequently sacrificed, interrupting the ever-present singing of the cicadas and competing with the exuberant voices and cheerful clamour of the initiates. The culmination of this sonic extravaganza must have been the procession of the nineteenth day of Boedromion (see below), one of the most remarkable religious events of the ancient world. Dressed in festal clothes,[15] crowned with wreaths, and holding great torches, the initiates, led by the youthful sonic god Iacchus and the members of the Eleusinian priestly personnel and sacred families (*gene*) of Kerykes and Eumolpidae, left Athens and, following the Sacred Way (*Hiera Hodos*), marched to Eleusis singing and rejoicing. Iacchus was the personification of the shouting and the enthusiasm which characterized the procession from Athens to Eleusis (Deubner 1932: 73). The name of the god derives from the Greek verb *iaccheō* or *iacchō* meaning 'to shout, to raise a cry, to mourn, to bewail' and it is used in the Homeric Hymn to Demeter (20) to describe Persephone's sonic reaction to her abduction by Hades.

The outer court of the sanctuary at Eleusis was not reached until midnight because many stops had to be made on the way before the altars, shrines and sanctuaries which flanked the *Hiera Hodos*. In fact, festive music, singing and joyous human exclamations were so closely identified with the festive processions from and to Eleusis that quite often they went unnoted in our primary evidence. By contrast, the absence of these

---

15 Contra Bremmer (2014: 17), who thinks that the initiates would wear less glamorous clothing if they were to dedicate them to the temple at the end of the initiatory rites.

jubilant sonic settings is often remarked upon and interpreted as a major sign of disruption in the order of the Greek cultic cosmos.

Take the procession of 407 BCE, for example, which, according to Plutarch (*Alcibiades* 34.3–7), was led by Alcibiades, the well-known fifth century BCE Athenian statesman, who also faced accusations of profaning the Mysteries of Eleusis during a drinking party (*symposium*). As Spartan garrisons had been placed on the way to Eleusis right after the fortification of Deceleia, 'the festivities conducted by the sea lacked splendour'. This effectively meant that sacrifices (*thysiae*), choral dances (*choreiae*) and many of the sacred ceremonies (*polla ton drōmenon*) usually held on the road, when the Iacchus procession was conducted forth from Athens to Eleusis, had out of necessity been omitted. Regardless, Alcibiades, along with the infantry, decided to escort the procession headed by the god Iacchus past the enemy by land in a decorous and silent way (*en kosmō kai meta siōpēs*). Not only did Agis, the Spartan king, keep quiet out of respect for the silent solemn spectacle (*theama semnon kai theoprepes*) but Alcibiades himself was heralded by his friends as a Hierophant and Mystagogue, two of the most prominent sacred officials of the festival who, respectively, revealed the sacred things (*hiera*) to the initiands (*mystae*) and led them to their initiation.

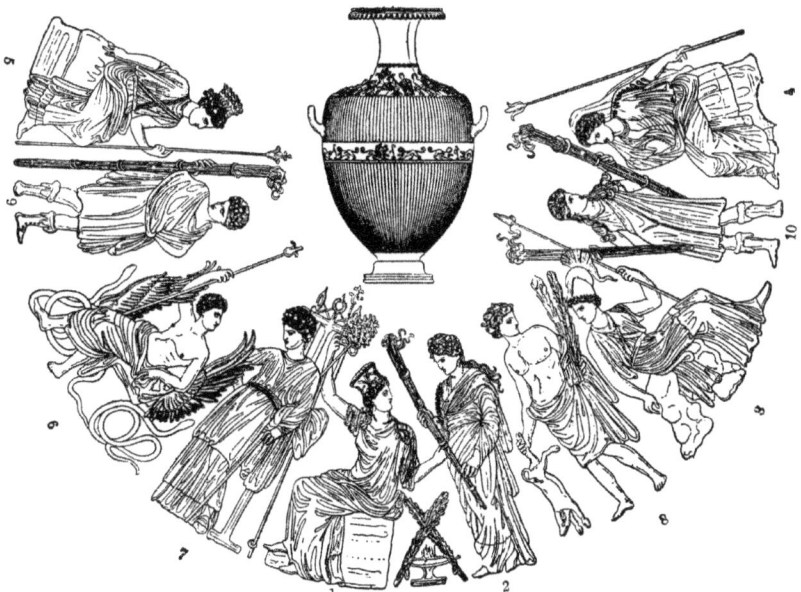

Figure 7.1 Drawing of a hydria (the 'Regina Vasorum') from Cumae, now in the Hermitage Museum, Saint Petersburg. The hydria portrays Iacchus (no. 9) and other Eleusinian deities and members of the priestly personnel. Drawing by author.

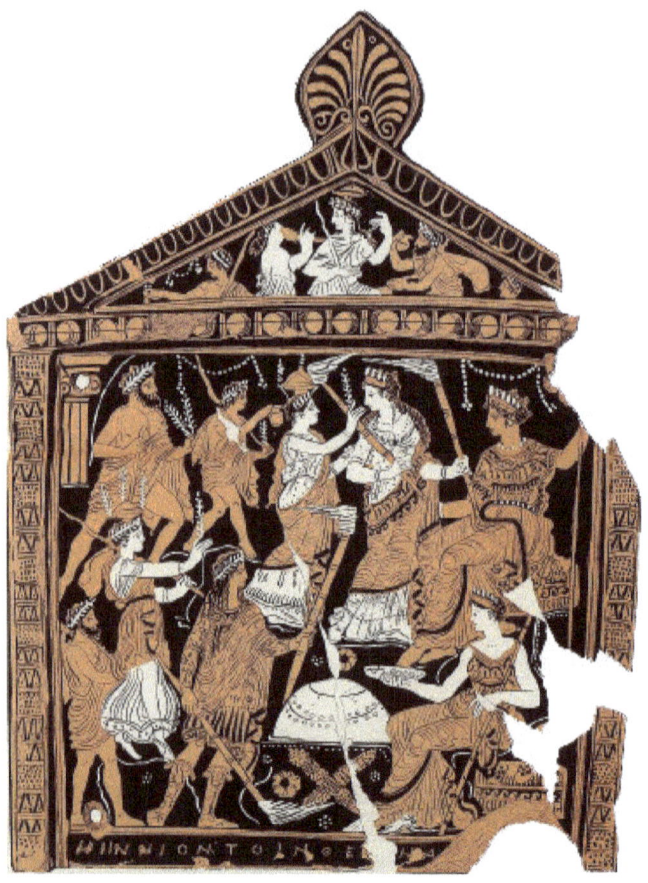

Figure 7.2 The Ninnion Tablet dated to approximately 370 BCE, now in the National Archaeological Museum, Athens. The votive tablet is made of clay and depicts, at bottom left of centre, a figure usually identified (by his ceremonial attire) as Iacchus leading a procession of initiates. The group of initiates and leading deities is received by the presiding deities of the Mysteries, Demeter and Kore, who are portrayed seated on the right-hand side of the relief. After Andreas N. Skias *Archaiologike Ephemeris* 1901: pinax 1.

In that instance it was silence that is marked as out of the ordinary, since it has replaced the vociferous Iacchus song (see below), the joyous choral dances (*choriae*) and many of the communal happenings that were normally at the heart of the auditory aesthetics of the Eleusinian procession. By conducting the Iacchus procession in a shroud of stillness, Alcibiades altered the semantics of the superimposed festive frugality, extending the mystique of the things that were not allowed to be seen, heard and done (*arrhēta* or *aporrhēta*, as part of the secret segment of initiatory rites which should not be divulged or else could not be communicated) to the public part of the ceremony. The solemn substitution of sound with silence transformed a ritual and therefore repetitive event into an extraordinarily politically charged protest. However, in order to properly appreciate the ingenuity of this substitution, we need to remind ourselves of how loud and festive the Iacchus procession would have been under normal political circumstances.

THE IACCHUS PROCESSION

On the day of the Mysteries known as *eikas*, i.e. 'the twentieth day',[16] an elaborate procession, with the priestesses of Eleusis in the lead, would escort the *hiera* from the Athenian Eleusinion, through the Agora, to the Dipylon and the temple of Iacchus, the Iaccheion, and then back to Eleusis (Plutarch, *Aristophanes and Menander* 27). In the Iaccheion they would find Iacchus in the form of his wooden statue. The youthful god, often depicted holding torches and wearing hunting boots (Figures 7.1 and 7.2), would lead the *mystae* to their final destination, the Eleusinian Telesterion (the Eleusinian initiation chamber, Figure 7.3).[17] According to Pausanias' *Description of Greece* (1.2.4, 1.37.4), the statue was made by the Athenian sculptor Praxiteles. That Iacchus' statue was perceived as the earthly

---

16 The nineteenth of Beodromion was called εἰκάς (= twentieth) because Greeks used to count the beginning of a day from sunset onwards. The procession would reach Eleusis towards the evening of the nineteenth; i.e. at the start of the twentieth day. This is at least the explanation given by Mylonas (1961: 256, n.151). Clinton (1986: 70) and Mansfield (1985: 434–437) argue in favour of two separate ephebic processions, one that would escort the *hiera* back to Eleusis on the nineteenth of Boedromion, and one other that would escort Iacchus' statue and the *mystae* to Eleusis the next day, that is on the twentieth of Boedromion. Graf (1996: 62–63) argues convincingly enough that such a hypothesis presents some serious logistic and textual problems. Mylonas' thesis is not discussed by Graf. More on the debate in Parker (2005: 348).

17 On Iacchus' iconographical physiognomy see for instance the relief hydria from Cumae (Figure 7.1), known otherwise as Regina Vasorum (Clinton 1992: 79, fig. III. 9; now in the Hermitage Museum, Saint Petersburg) and the Ninnion pinax from Eleusis (Figure 7.2, now in the National Archaeological Museum, Athens 11036); Mylonas (1961: fig. 88, and 213–221). Cf. also Graf (1974: 46–50) and Clinton (1992: 90–95; Clinton 2007: 349–350, figs. 22.3 and 22.2 respectively). Cf. also Jiménez San Cristóbal (2012): 125–135.

manifestation of the god is evident from the kind of treatment it received: it was crowned with a wreath of myrtle and was carried in a carriage, an honour denied to the *mystae* and reserved only for the priestly personnel and the god himself. The Iacchagōgos, the god's priest, would take his place with the god's image at the head of the procession, which followed Demeter on the road to Eleusis (*Hiera Hodos*) amidst much sacred exhilaration and festive singing.[18] Judging from epigraphic evidence and the comic version of the song found in Aristophanes' *Frogs* (314–413), while on their way, the *mystae* would sing the Iacchus-song, which would invoke the god to accompany them. They would often stop briefly to get some rest from the wearisome journey and perform sacrifices, choral songs and various *drōmena* (Plutarch's *Alcibiades* 34, 3–5; *Inscriptiones Graecae* II²1078, 29).

In historical times, it was believed that Iacchus' epiphany was perceived by both Greeks and Persians in the course of the naval battle of Salamis (480 BCE). The story is preserved by both Herodotus (*Histories* 8.65) and Plutarch (*Themistocles* 15.1). In Herodotus' longer and more detailed account, Iacchus' epiphany is perceived by two exiles in the court of the Persian king: the Spartan Demaratus and the Athenian Dicaeus. Both witnesses are familiar with the cultural conventions of the Great Mysteria and Iacchus' procession as one of its main sonic highlights. In other words, both men were able to recognise not only the natural sonic component of the procession but also its cultural significance. It is no surprise, then, that they are the ones who are able to disambiguate a 'cloud of dust, such as might have been raised by an army of thirty thousand men on the march, coming from the direction of Eleusis', and interpret it as part of that procession. Dicaeus even thought he recognised the Iacchus song and, given that there were no men left in Athens after the evacuation, he concluded that the voice they heard was clearly not human but divine. Shortly afterwards, we are told, this cloud of dust rose high into the air and drifted away towards Salamis, something that Dicaeus explains as a divine sign of the destruction of the Persian fleet.

In Plutarch's shorter version, 'a great light flashed out (*phōs eklampsai mega*) from Eleusis, and a sound and a voice (*ēchon de kai phōnēn*) filled the

---

18 Pausanius (1.24) mentions a statue of Iacchus by Praxiteles. Evidence that the procession to Eleusis is following the steps of Demeter, or else that Demeter was imagined to accompany the chorus to their pilgrimage, is provided in Aristophanes' *Frogs*, 384ff.: the chorus invokes Demeter to stand by their side (συμπαραστάτει) and in 399–400 they point out that Iacchus is following Demeter: δεῦρο συνακολούθει πρὸς τὴν θεόν.

Thracian field right down to the sea, as though coming from a large body of men escorting the mystic Iacchus (*ton mystikon eksagōnton Iacchon*) in a procession. Then, out of the shouting throng, a cloud (*nephos*) seemed slowly to rise up from the land and then to come down.' It is as if in 480 BCE the gods decided to take part themselves in the festival that the Athenians had cancelled because of Persian Wars. Iacchus manifested himself by an auditory epiphany, a reverberating sound alluding to the god's true acoustic nature.[19]

More than a century later, when Athens had yielded to the all-conquering Macedon, a Macedonian garrison happened to be instituted in Athens on the *eikas*, the day of the boisterous Iacchus' procession (*eksagōgē*). According to Plutarch's *Phocion* (28.1–3), the Athenians found this coincidence particularly painful. Looking back at previous glamorous celebrations of the Mysteries with nostalgia, they lamented the substitution of the jubilant clamour of the procession of the initiates with the Macedonian marching and interpreted it as a sign of divine indifference and neglect. Unlike what happened in Salamis, the gods had now allowed for the profanation of the Mysteries:

> For of old the mystic visions (*mysticas opseis*) and voices (*phōnas*) were granted to them in the midst of their most glorious successes, and brought amazement (*ekplēksis*) and awe (*thambos*) upon their enemies; but now, while in the same sacred ceremonies, the gods looked down with indifference upon the most grievous woes of Greece, and the profanation of the season which had been most sweet and holy in their eyes.

Dio Chrysostom (*Orations* 12.33) refers also to 'mystic visions and mystic voices' (*polla men horōnta mystica theamata, pollōn de akouonta toioutōn phōnōn*) but it is unclear which mysteries he has in mind. The ritual seating (*thronismos*) of the initiate mentioned in the same passage is attested for the Corybantic rites (Plato, *Euthydemus* 277d), while it has also been conjectured for the Kabeiric mysteries in Samothrace by Nock (1941: 577–578). A form of *thronismos* is also attested in Apuleius' *Metamorphoses* 11 and may have been a constituent ritual element in Eleusis, if we are to read lines 250–255 from Aristophanes' *Clouds* as a parody of the Eleusinian Mysteries.

---

19 Deubner (1932: 73), who compares *Iacchus* to another personification of a song, that of *Hymenaios*.

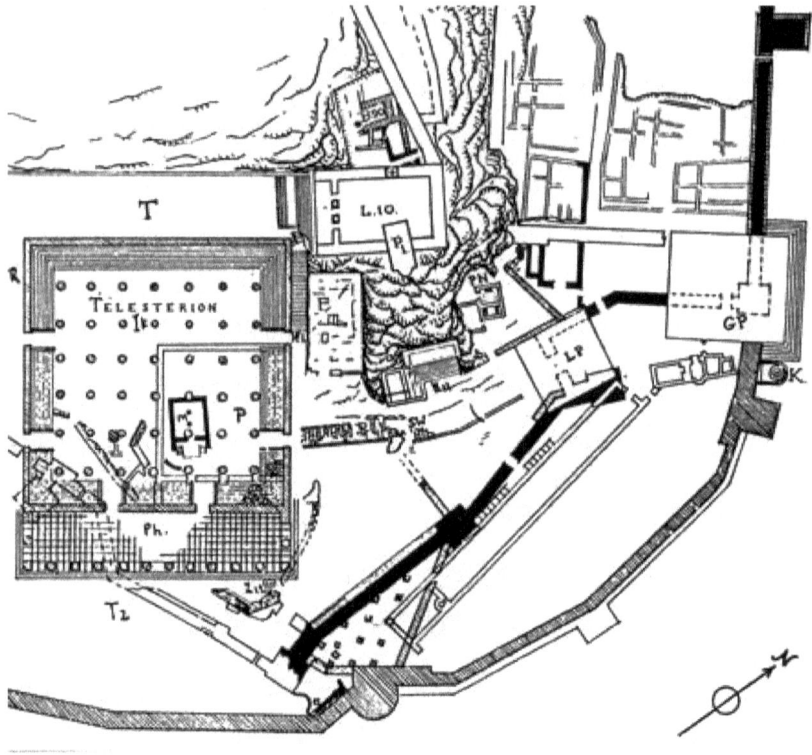

Figure 7.3 Map of the Eleusinian sanctuary. After Mylonas (1947).

ELEUSINIAN SOUNDSCAPE: THE SECRET SEGMENT

Mystic visions and voices are placed on an equal footing in Plutarch's passage quoted above. Neither is deemed more important than the other; instead, they are both situated in the centre of the multisensory initiatory experience in Eleusis. However, testimonies that report the extraordinary acoustic environs of Eleusis are, at best, commented on *en passant* in the scholarly literature and, at worst, are completely ignored. I have already mentioned the ephemerality of, and the limited amount of, evidence regarding the sonic settings of the part of the festival that took place in the Telesterion as possible causes of the scholarly disinterest in the sonorous aspect of the Eleusinian rites. Nonetheless, the scholarly reluctance to see the Eleusinian initiatory rites as a multisensory event may also be the result of a projection of Christian ideas about the pre-eminence of intellectual stimulation over the sensory back onto the ancient world. Michael Cosmopoulos, for example, in his recent book on Bronze Age Eleusis, interprets Aristotle's laying of emphasis on the initiatory experience and using the infinitive *pathein*, i.e. 'suffering' (Fr. 15 Rose)[20] as follows: 'This would suggest that the experience of the initiates was spiritual and did not rely on the world of the senses'. However, to my mind Aristotle's privileging of *pathein* (i.e. acquiring knowledge via suffering) over *mathein* (i.e. acquiring knowledge via cognitive processes) equates with an emphasis on the embodied and ensounded experience of the initiates rather than their intellectual processing of the auditory and visual stimuli to which they were exposed in the process of the initiation.

As I have argued before (Petridou 2013), there are numerous theoretical reconstructions of the exact nature of the mythical events dramatised for the eyes and the ears of the *mystae*, but, essentially, they can be summarised as follows: we can either assume with scholars like Nicolas Richardson (1974) that Demeter's sufferings *were simply narrated to the initiates at some stage during the sacred rites*, and that even if there was some sort of re-enactment of the mythical events, it would have been of a more formal and symbolic nature; or we can look at other students of the Eleusinian *mystēria*, such as George Mylonas, Kevin Clinton, Walter Burkert and Christiane Sourvinou-Inwood, who maintain that the re-enactment of the divine sufferings was of a mimetic nature, and that both priestly personnel and initiates participated in the ritual. Richardson (1974: 24-25) builds his main argument around the following passage from Isocrates' *Panygericus* (28–29), in which we are told about Demeter's gifts to the Athenians, gifts 'of which only the initiated may hear':

> Now, first of all, that which was the first necessity of man's nature was provided by our city; for even though the story has taken the form of a myth, yet it deserves to be told again. When Demeter came to our land, in her wandering after the rape of Kore, and, being moved to kindness towards our ancestors by services which may not be told save to her initiates, gave these two gifts, the greatest in the world – the fruits of the earth, which have enabled us to rise above the life of the beasts, and the holy rite which inspires in those who partake of it sweeter hopes regarding both the end of life and all eternity, our city was not only so beloved of the gods but also so

---

20 Cosmopoulos (2015: 15). Aristotle Fr. 15 Rose: 'thus, Aristotle has it that the initiants must not learn something in particular, but suffer and being psychologically predisposed', as quoted by Synesius Dion. 10.271 Krab. (cf. Dio Chrysostom, *Orations* 12.33f).

devoted to mankind that, having been endowed with these great blessings, she did not begrudge them to the rest of the world, but shared with all men what she had received. The mystic rite we continue even now, each year, to reveal to the initiates; and as for the fruits of the earth, our city has, in a word, instructed the world in their uses, their cultivation, and the benefits derived from them. (transl. George Norlin, Loeb Classical Library)

The passage implies that Demeter's wanderings across the earth during her search for her daughter, and the benefactions the Athenians received from the goddess pertaining to both agriculture and afterlife, were part of the Sacred Discourse (*hieros logos*) of the cult (Henrichs 2003; Bremmer 2014). It is indeed possible that the initiates heard an elaboration, and/or an exegesis, of the story of the suffering goddesses as part of their initiation. Although this chapter aims at raising awareness of the richness of the Eleusinian soundscape by focusing on sound and hearing, we ought to be careful and not attempt to reduce a multisensory experience to one or the other sensory register. The fact that the orator refers to things that only those initiated could hear does not necessarily mean that the *mystae* were only listening to sacred words spoken. Isocrates simply makes a self-reference and reminds his initiated listeners why he does not go into depth about the Mysteries: so he would not commit sacrilege by revealing anything to non-initiates. He only speaks of listening because this is the only possible danger he faces: revealing the Mysteries by uttering something inappropriate. As expected, not much is known about what constituted the things that should not be divulged or else cannot be communicated (*arrhēta* or *aporrhēta*) of the Mysteries, what percentage of those forbidden things pertained to hearing and what to vision. Yet, we can, with some degree of certainty, assume that those who divulged the Mysteries in 415, according to Pseudo-Lysias (6.51), 'not only did they parody the rites, they also spoke the secrets'.[21]

However, there are other sources which may suggest that the secret segment of the initiation was also an opulent audial setting. The Stoic Cleanthes (*Stoicorum Veterum Frangmenta* 1.538), for example, implies that a special kind of sacred semiology and an exegetical exposition of the secret names of the presiding deities may have been employed in the

---

21 Pseudo-Lysias 6 is a prosecution speech against Andocides IV, accusing him of both mutilating herms and parodying in the mysteries. MacDowell (1962) argues that the speech is genuine, not a later pamphlet, but spoken by Meletus II, Epichares, or Agyrrhius – and most likely by Meletus II. Cf. also Marr (1971).

initiatory chambers of Eleusinian Telesterion, when he speaks of gods as mystic shapes (*mystica schemata*) and sacred invocations (*klēseis hieras*) in the context of mystic rites of Eleusis (Scade 2017: 208). Moreover, Clement of Alexandria (*Protrepticos* 2.12), who was born a pagan and then converted to Christianity, speaks of mournful sounds as being part of the *drama mystikon*: 'Demeter and Persephone have come to be the subject of a mystic drama, and Eleusis celebrates with torches the rape of the daughter and the sorrowful wandering of the mother.'

If indeed a ritual search was conducted to find Demeter's lost offspring, we can safely assume that acoustically it would have been accompanied by loud ritual lamentations for the lost Kore. Julius Firmicus Maternus (*De Errore Profanarum Religionum* 22.1), who wrote in the reign of Constantine I (306 to 337 CE), if indeed he refers to the initiatory rites of Eleusis, may be providing us with a sonic snippet of the initiatory ceremony, when he maintains that:

> On a certain night an image is placed supine on a bed, and is rhythmically and profusely lamented. Then, when they have satiated themselves with feigned lamentation, light is brought in. The priest anoints the throats of all who were weeping. And the priest murmurs slowly: 'take courage, initiates, for the god is saved, and you will have out of suffering salvation'.[22]

It is not clear though, whether these lamentations were produced by the initiates or members of the priestly personnel who may have enacted the ritual search of the mother for her daughter. A fragment of Apollodorus of Athens (*Die Fragmente der griechischen Historiker* 244F 110b) also supports this idea of boisterous and sonically charged ritual search being in the centre of the *drama mystikon*. In particular, Apollodorus thinks that a gong-like sound and solemn invocations were heard at some point of the ritual search for the Kore in Eleusis: 'When Kore is being called up the hierophant strikes the bronze gong. They also strike the cymbal, when a Laconian king dies.' Sourvinou-Inwood (2003: 33) rightly thinks that such a solemn invocation would have been most appropriate at some climactic point in the search:

> a solemn invocation of Kore alone would make excellent ritual sense as part of the search: after it had run its course, and before the deity was 'found', the

---

22 This is, of course, only if we assume that this specific part of *On the Errors of the Profane Religion* refers to the Great Mysteria of Eleusis.

invocation would have taken place, with the hierophant sounding the gong. Solemn invocations, though common and by no means limited to advent festivals – nevertheless had a special place in both, since both focused on the deity's arrival, which was the objective of an invocation.

On the other hand, Hippolytus of Rome (*Refutation of all Heresies* 5.8.40) quotes a Naassenian, a Gnostic who identifies all the mysteries with Gnostic Christianity and claims that he knew of the exact content of the secret invocations that were heard during the first stage of initiation, the *myēsis*: 'At night in Eleusis the hierophant with much fire performing the great and unmistakable mysteries shouts out loud, saying: "the mistress has given birth to a sacred boy, Brimo to Brimos".' Nonetheless, the same author (*Refutation of all Heresies* 5.8.39) postulates a much more modest affair for the culmination of the second and higher stage of the initiation, the *epopteia*: '… the Athenians performing the Eleusinian initiations and displaying to the *epoptai* the great and marvellous and perfect epoptic mystery, in silence, a reaped ear of corn'.

Lactantius (*Divine Institutes* 23) supports the idea of a raucous ritual search being at the heart of the Eleusinian sacred drama and focuses again on its climax. He postulates that the ritual search ended with the throwing away of the torches in an atmosphere of sonic exultation with the initiates (and perhaps also the members of the priestly personnel) congratulating one another.[23] A passage from Stobaeus (in which he quotes Plutarch; Stobaeus IV.52.49 = Plut. Fr. 178) sheds light on the emotive responses of those partaking in the ritual search and adds mystic choruses (*choreias*), voices (*phōnas*) and solemn utterances (*semnōtētas akousmatōn hierōn*) to the acoustic gamut of the secret segment of Eleusis.

In a recently published article (2013), Richard Seaford has made an appealing suggestion: 'the chorus of mystic initiates, in imagining themselves as coexistent with the cosmos as they prefigured their eternal solidarity, provided both for Platonic philosophy and (differently) for the polis a transcendent model of happy cohesion'. In the same article, Seaford discusses the singing and dancing of the initiates in the course of the Iacchus procession, as well as the dancing at Eleusis around the Kallichoron well mentioned by Pausanias (1.38.6). He rightly claims that the happy chorus of initiates in Aristophanes' *Frogs* alludes to 'the exhilarated solidarity of the processional singing and dancing initiates', which 'can be publicly

---

23 *His etiam Cereris simile mysterium est, in quo facibus accensis per noctem Proserpina inquitur et ea inventua ritus omnis gratulatione et taedarum iactatione finitur.*

displayed without revealing what was revealed only in the rite of passage'. It is this happy mystic chorus of initiates that provides the bridge between the secret and the public segments of the festival, since, as Seaford reminds us, the phrase 'to dance out the mysteries (*eksorcheisthai ta mystēria*)' is used quite frequently to describe the Eleusinian initiatory rites (e.g.: Lucian, *De saltatione* 15; Alciphron 3.72; Achilles Tatius 4.8; *Oxyrhynchus Papyri* 411.25). This image of the mystic chorus dancing in exultation takes us back to Ingold's idea about the ensounded body, the body that, although firmly grounded, is launched into the sound like a kite in the sky, and makes us lament even more the lack of additional concrete evidence about Eleusis' sonorous culture.

Simultaneously, it raises the following question: if indeed sound was so multifaceted and prominent in Eleusis, why were the Eleusinian Mysteries so closely identified with the proverbial silence that shrouded the *arrhēta* or *aporrhēta*? Bremmer (2014: 1–20), in his recent description of the Eleusinian Mysteries, shows amply enough that the answer lies with the Platonic reception of the Eleusinian imagery and terminology, and the subsequent adoption of Plato's Eleusis by the Christian authors and the literati of the so-called second sophistic. To take the famous second century CE orator Aelius Aristides as an example, he, like many of his contemporaries, made use of mysteric silence and *aposiōpēsis* as a discursive tool, which allowed him to make claims of possessing the ultimate truth in both religious and medical matters without having to go the extra mile of actually providing any proof for his claims (van Nuffelen 2007: 21; 2011).[24] Nonetheless, it is extremely important to clarify here that using mysteric silence as a rhetorical tool is not an act of irreverence, nor does it preclude a simultaneous expression of genuine religious fervour. Plutarch uses the same technique in his *De defectu oraculorum, De facie, De Iside*, certain parts of the *Questiones Conviviales*, and elsewhere (Montiglio 1984; van Nuffelen 2007). And here we return to the idea of how resonant the Eleusinian Mysteria were with both contemporaries and posterity. Instead of lamenting the lost natural and cultural components of the Eleusinian soundscape, we should focus on its resounding nature. Through thousands of years and through hundreds of authors, both ancient and modern, Eleusis still rings a bell.

---

24 I am indebted to Peter Van Nuffelen for sharing with me a copy of the article and his thoughts on the subject. On silence in general as a powerful rhetorical tool, see Montiglio (2000: esp. 116–137). On secrecy and concealment in the religious history of the Mediterranean, see Kippenberg and Stroumsa (1995).

REFERENCES

Athanassakis, A. N. 1976. 'Music and Ritual in Primitive Eleusis', *Platon* 28: 86–105.
Bowden, H. 2010. *Mystery Cults of the Ancient World*. Princeton: Princeton University Press.
Bremmer, J. N. 2014. *Initiation into the Mysteries of the Ancient World*. Berlin and New York: De Gruyter. https://doi.org/10.1515/9783110299557
Burkert, W. 1983. *Homo Necans: The Anthropology of Ancient Greek Sacrificial Ritual and Myth*. Berkeley: University of California Press.
Burkert, W. 1987. *Ancient Mystery Cults*. Cambridge, MA: Harvard University Press.
Calame, C. 2001. *Choruses of Young Women in Ancient Greece: Their Morphology, Religious Role, and Social Function*. [English trans. of *Les Chœurs de jeunes filles en Grèce archaïque*, 2 vols. (Rome, 1977) by D. Collins and J. Orion], 2nd edn. Lanham, MD: Rowman & Littlefield Publishers.
Clinton, K. 1986. 'The Author of the Homeric Hymn to Demeter', *Opuscula Atheniensia* 16: 43–49.
Clinton, K. 1992. *Myth and Cult*. Stockholm: Svenska Institutet i Athen.
Clinton, K. 1993. 'The Sanctuary of Demeter and Kore at Eleusis' in N. Marinatos and R. Hägg (eds), *Greek Sanctuaries*. London: Routledge. pp. 110–124.
Clinton, K. 2003. 'Stages of Initiation in the Eleusinian and Samothracian Mysteries' in Cosmopoulos (2003: 50–78).
Clinton, K. 2005. 'Pigs in Greek Rituals' in R. Hägg and B. Alroth (eds), *Greek Sacrificial Ritual: Olympian and Chthonian*. Stockholm: Svenska Institutet i Athen. pp. 167–179.
Clinton, K. 2005–2008. *Eleusis, the Inscriptions on Stone: Documents of the Sanctuary of the Two Goddesses and Public Documents of the Deme* (2 vols). Athens: Archaeological Society at Athens.
Clinton, K. 2007. 'The Mysteries of Demeter and Kore' in D. Ogden (ed.), *A Companion to Greek Religion*. London and New York: Wiley-Blackwell. pp. 342–356.
Cosmopoulos, M. B. (ed.) 2003. *Greek Mysteries: The Archaeology and Ritual of Ancient Greek Secret Cults*. London and New York: Routledge.
Cosmopoulos, M. B. 2015. *Bronze Age Eleusis and the Origins of the Eleusinian Mysteries*. Cambridge: Cambridge University Press. https://doi.org/10.1017/CBO9780511820700
Deubner, L. 1932. *Attische Feste*. Berlin: H. Keller.
Dickie, M. W. 2004. 'Priestly Proclamations and Sacred Laws', *Classical Quarterly* 54: 579–591. https://doi.org/10.1093/clquaj/bmh059
Dover, K. 1993. *Aristophanes' Frogs. Edited with and Introduction and Commentary*. Oxford: Clarendon Press.
Dowden, K. 1980. 'Grades in the Eleusinian Mysteries', *Revue de l'histoire des Religions* 197: 409–27. https://doi.org/10.3406/rhr.1980.4993
Ekroth, G. 2002. *The Sacrificial Rituals of Greek Hero Cults in the Archaic to Early Hellenistic Periods*. Liège: Centre International d'Étude de la Religion Grecque Antique.
Ekroth, G. 2007. 'Meat in Ancient Greece: Sacrificial, Sacred, or Secular', *Food and History* 5.1: 249–72.

Ekroth, G. 2008. 'Burnt, Cooked or Raw? Divine and Human Culinary Desires at Greek Animal Sacrifice' in E. Stavrianopoulou, A. Michaels, and C. Ambos (eds), *Transformations in Sacrificial Practices.* Berlin and Münster: LIT Verlag Berlin-Münster. pp. 87–112.

Emerit, S., Perrot, S., and Vincent, A. (eds). 2015. *Le paysage sonore de l'Antiquité Méthodologie, historiographie et perspectives.* Paris: Institut français d'archéologie orientale.

Gaifmann, M. 2012. *Aniconism in Greek Antiquity.* Oxford: Oxford University Press.

Graf, F. 1974. *Eleusis und die orphische Dictung Athens in vorhellenistischer Zeit, RGVV* 33. Berlin: De Gruyter.

Graf, F. 1996. '*Pompai* in Greece: Some Considerations about Space and Ritual in the Greek Polis' in R. Hägg (ed.), *The Role of Religion in the Early Greek Polis.* Stockholm: Svenska Institutet i Athen. pp. 55–65.

Graf, F. 2003. 'Lesser Mysteries—Not Less Mysterious' in Cosmopoulos (2003: 241–62).

Guarducci, M. 1982. 'Le Rane di Aristofane e la topografia ateniese', *Studi in onore di Aristide Colonna* (Perugia): 167–172.

Henrichs, A. 2003. 'Hieroi Logoi and Hierai Bibloi: The (Un)written Margins of the Sacred in Ancient Greece', *Harvard Studies in Classical Philology* 101: 207–266.

Hitch, S. and Rutherford, I. (eds). 2013. *Animal Sacrifice in the Ancient Greek World.* Cambridge: Cambridge University Press.

Hooker, G. T. W. 1960. 'The Topography of the Frogs', *Journal of Hellenic Studies* 80: 112–117. https://doi.org/10.2307/628380

Ingold, T. 2000. *The Perception of the Environment: Essays in Livelihood, Dwelling and Skill.* London: Routledge. https://doi.org/10.4324/9780203466025

Ingold, T. 2007. 'Against Soundscape' in E. Carlyle (ed.), *Autumn Leaves: Sound and the Environment in Artistic Practice.* Paris: Double Entendre. pp. 10–13.

Jiménez San Cristóbal, A. I. 2012. 'Iacchus in Plutarch' in L. Roig Lanzillotta and I. Muñoz Gallarte (eds), *Plutarch in the Religious and Philosophical Discourse of Late Antiquity.* Leiden: Brill. pp. 125–135.

Kippenberg, H. G., and Stroumsa, G. G. (eds). 1995. *Secrecy and Concealment: Studies in the History of Mediterranean and Near Eastern Religions.* Leiden: Brill.

Kubatzki, J. 2016. 'Music in Rites. Some Thoughts about the Function of Music in Ancient Greek Cults', *eTopoi, Journal for Ancient Studies* 5: 1–17.

MacDowell, D. M. (ed.) 1962. *Andokides: On the Mysteries.* Oxford Clarendon Press.

Mansfield, J. M. 1985. *The Robe of Athena and the Panathenaic 'Peplos'*, dissertation, University of California, Berkeley.

Marr, J. L. 1971. 'Andocides' Part in the Mysteries and Hermae Affairs 415 BC', *Classical Quarterly* 21: 326–338. https://doi.org/10.1017/S0009838800033474

Montiglio, S. 1984. *I silenzi di Plutarcho*, dissertation, Pavia.

Montiglio, S. 2000. *Silence in the Land of Logos.* Princeton: Princeton University Press.

Mylonas, G. E. 1947. 'Eleusis and the Eleusinian Mysteries', *The Classical Journal* 43: 130–146.

Mylonas, G. E. 1961. *Eleusis and the Eleusinian Mysteries.* Princeton: Princeton University Press.

Naiden, F. S. 2013. *Smoke Signals for the Gods: Ancient Greek Sacrifice from the Archaic through the the Roman Periods.* Oxford: Oxford University Press.

Nock, A. D. 1941. 'A Cabiric Rite', *American Journal of Archaeology* 45: 577–81.
Parker, R. 2005. *Polytheism and Society at Athens*, Oxford: Oxford University Press.
Pavolini, C. 2015. 'La Musica e il Culto di Cibele nell'occidente Romano', *ArchCl* LXVI: 345–375.
Petridou, G. 2013. 'Blessed is he, who has seen…: The Power of Ritual Viewing and Ritual Framing in Eleusis' in S. Blundell, D. Cairns and N. Rabinowitz (eds), *Vision and Viewing in Ancient Greece*, Helios 40: 309–341. https://doi.org/10.1353/hel.2013.0015
Petridou, G. 2015. *Divine Epiphany in Greek Literature and Culture*. Oxford: Oxford University Press. https://doi.org/10.1093/acprof:oso/9780198723929.001.0001
Richardson, N. J. 1974. *The Homeric Hymn to Demeter*. Oxford: Oxford University Press.
Rosa, H. 2012. *Weltbeziehungen im Zeitalter der Beschleunigun*. Berlin: Suhrkamp.
Rosa, H. 2014. 'Resonanz statt Entfremdung, Zehn Thesen wider die Steigerungslogik der Moderne' in L. Kirschenmann and F. Wittmann (eds), *Zeitwohlstand*. Leipzig: Konzeptwerk Neue Ökonomie. pp. 62–73.
Rosa, H. 2016. *Resonanz: Eine Soziologie der Weltbeziehung*. Berlin: Suhrkamp Verlag.
Samuels, D. W., Meintjes, L., Ochoa A. M., and Procello, T. 2010. 'Soundscapes: Towards a Sounded Anthropology', *Annual Review of Anthropology* 39: 329–345. https://doi.org/10.1146/annurev-anthro-022510-132230
Scade, P. R. 2017. 'Music and the Soul in Stoicism' in R. Seaford, J. Wilkins and M. Wright (eds), *Selfhood and the Soul: Essays on Ancient Thought and Literature in Honour of Christopher Gill*. Oxford: Oxford University Press. pp. 197–218. https://doi.org/10.1093/acprof:oso/9780198777250.003.0011
Seaford, R. A. S. 2013. 'The Politics of the Mystic Chorus' in J. Billings, F. Budelmann and F. Macintosh (eds), *Choruses, Ancient and Modern*. Oxford: Oxford University Press. pp. 261–280. https://doi.org/10.1093/acprof:oso/9780199670574.003.0016
Simms, R. 1990. 'Myesis, Telete, and Mysteria', *Greek, Roman, and Byzantine Studies* 31: 183–195.
Sourvinou-Inwood, C. 1997. 'Reconstructing Change: Ideology and the Eleusinian Mysteries' in M. Golden and P. Toohey (eds), *Inventing Ancient Culture*. London: Routledge. pp. 132–164.
Sourvinou-Inwood, C. 2003. 'Festival and Mysteries: Aspects of the Eleusinian Cult' in Cosmopoulos (2003: 25–49).
Sourvinou-Inwood, C. 2006. 'The Priesthoods of the Eleusinian Cult of Demeter and Kore', *Thesaurus Cultuum et Rituum Antiquorum* 5: 60–65.
Tierney, M. 1934/5. 'The *Parodos* in Aristophanes' Frogs', *Proceedings of the Royal Irish Academy* 42: 199–218.
van Nuffelen, P. 2007. 'Words of Truth: Mystical Silence as a Philosophical and Rhetorical Tool in Plutarch', *Hermathena* 182: 9–39.
van Nuffelen, P. 2011. *Rethinking Gods: Philosophical Readings of Religion in the Post-Hellenistic Period*. Cambridge: Cambridge University Press.
West, M. L. 1992. *Ancient Greek Music*. Oxford: Clarendon Press.

Georgia Petridou is a Lecturer in Ancient Greek History at the University of Liverpool, UK. She is the author of *Divine Epiphany in Greek Literature and Culture* (Oxford University Press, 2015) and the co-editor of *Homo Patiens: Approaches to the Patient in the Ancient World* (with Chiara Thumiger; Brill, 2016) and *Beyond Priesthood: Religious Entrepreneurs and Innovators in the Imperial Era* (with Richard Gordon and Jörg Rüpke; De Gruyter, 2017). Her current research focuses on the intersections of ancient medicine and religion.

Chapter 8

North American Indigenous Song, the Sacred and the Senses

BYRON DUECK

Song plays a central role in many forms of North American Indigenous sacred observance. In the western Canadian city of Winnipeg, where I began ethnographic fieldwork in the early 2000s, two kinds of singing are especially important: drum song, which is heard in both traditional ceremonies and public performances, and gospel singing, widely performed at funerary wakes.

The most public contexts for drum song are powwows – large gatherings where it accompanies dancing in a range of traditional and neo-traditional styles. These events can be overwhelming for a first-time visitor. There is in the first place a profusion of things to see: dances in various genres bring several performers together at the centre of the arena, but although they wear similar kinds of regalia and dance in the same styles, both clothing and choreography are highly personalised, and there is a great deal of particularity to take in. Powwows are also aurally imposing: singers at northern events tend to perform with high, tensed voices and a wide vibrato, and they accompany themselves on impressively loud drums. In echoing arenas with the singing amplified through a large sound system, one can feel completely surrounded by the sound, with the drum in particular impacting not just the ears but the whole body.

Gospel singing is more subdued, especially when sung at wakes and funerals, its most important contexts of performance. I regularly attended such events in Winnipeg in 2002 and 2003, frequenting also a handful of coffeehouses where Indigenous gospel musicians met to sing in less serious circumstances. A range of singers from different communities and

Indigenous groups participated in the latter gatherings, where nearly anyone was welcome to participate. At one coffeehouse, I occasionally played bass with the band that accompanied the performers. In this role, I was struck by the distinctive rhythmic interpretations different singers brought to the same songs, and how these necessitated continual recalibrations on the part of the musicians performing with them. I also participated in drum singing from time to time – it was a regular activity at the urban powwow clubs I attended – and developed some familiarity with how it felt to perform in that style.

This chapter reflects on experiences of these two kinds of song to suggest some of the ways that sound, and especially music, shapes the experience of the sacred. It argues that music, by means of what I will call its mutable iconicity, is especially well suited to mediating sacred presences and processes. I also explore how musical practices assert and engender social difference: in the case of Indigenous song, this happens through not only the prominent use of distinctive languages, instruments, genres and styles of vocal production, but also the inclusive and participatory character of the contexts in which this music-making occurs.

DRUM SONG

Before European contact, the great majority of North American Indigenous music was song, often accompanied by percussion instruments such as drums and rattles (see Nettl 2001: 263–264; Diamond et al. 1994). Notwithstanding the active suppression of Indigenous traditions under colonialism, drum song persists in many Indigenous communities, and practices continue to emerge, circulate and be adopted, sometimes in places far from their point of origin, or where older traditions had nearly been extinguished.

In part thanks to revivals, drum song has a significant place in Winnipeg, a city with one of the largest populations of urban Indigenous people in North America. This heterogeneous population comprises Métis, Anishinaabe (Ojibwe), Cree, Oji-Cree, Dakota and Dene people, among others, with Northern Algonquians (Anishinaabe, Cree, Oji-Cree and Métis of related heritage) playing an especially prominent part in shaping contemporary Indigenous musical life. For this reason I will sometimes refer to 'Northern Algonquian' song and sacred observance, a term that has the advantage of highlighting their contributions to these practices, and the disadvantage of de-emphasising other groups, especially the Dakota, who have played a central role in preserving and disseminating drum song.

Drum song is most commonly performed by solo singers accompanying themselves on hand drums, or by drum groups consisting of several musicians seated around a large drum positioned with the skin facing upward. While drum songs employ special formal structures that reflect their Indigenous origins (see Levine and Nettl 2011), they are generally straightforward and readily learned by non-specialists. It is not unusual to hear children singing the same songs as adults, whether at social gatherings for young people or in public performance.

Drums are employed to do sacred work and are considered sacred themselves. On the one hand, they frequently accompany songs that address and invoke sacred beings, including Gichi Manidoo (Great Spirit), Makwa (Bear) and Ma'iingan (Wolf), to use the Anishinaabemowin (Ojibwe language) terms.[1] On the other, they are often understood to *have* spirits, and singers are careful to treat them with respect. That drums both have spirits and enable communication with them hints at some of the complex ways music mediates spiritual presences and processes, a topic addressed at greater length below.

Drum song is central to many sacred ceremonies. I will not say much about these events, in part because of concerns that publishing detailed accounts of them is disrespectful to the people and spirit beings who are present at them, and in part because it is considered problematic for non-Indigenous persons like me to seek advantage as brokers of ceremonial knowledge.[2] Accordingly, in what follows, I recount only information that is widely known, focusing for the most part on powwows, gatherings that incorporate sacred elements, but are nevertheless open to the public.[3]

Powwows are large gatherings where dancers in special regalia perform in a range of genres to music provided by drum groups (see Figure 8.1). The latter are ensembles comprising several drumming singers seated around a large drum positioned with skin facing upward (see Figure 8.2), sometimes with additional standing singers. A gendered division of musical labour, understood to be in keeping with tradition (see Browner 2002:

---

1 Ojibwe pronunciation and spelling vary widely; spelling here follows the *Ojibwe People's Dictionary* (University of Minnesota 2016).
2 This is not to say scholarly accounts of these ceremonies do not exist; see for instance Deloria (1929) or Bucko (1998).
3 On the powwow, see Browner (2002); Ellis et al. (2005); Scales (2007 and 2012); Levine (2013).

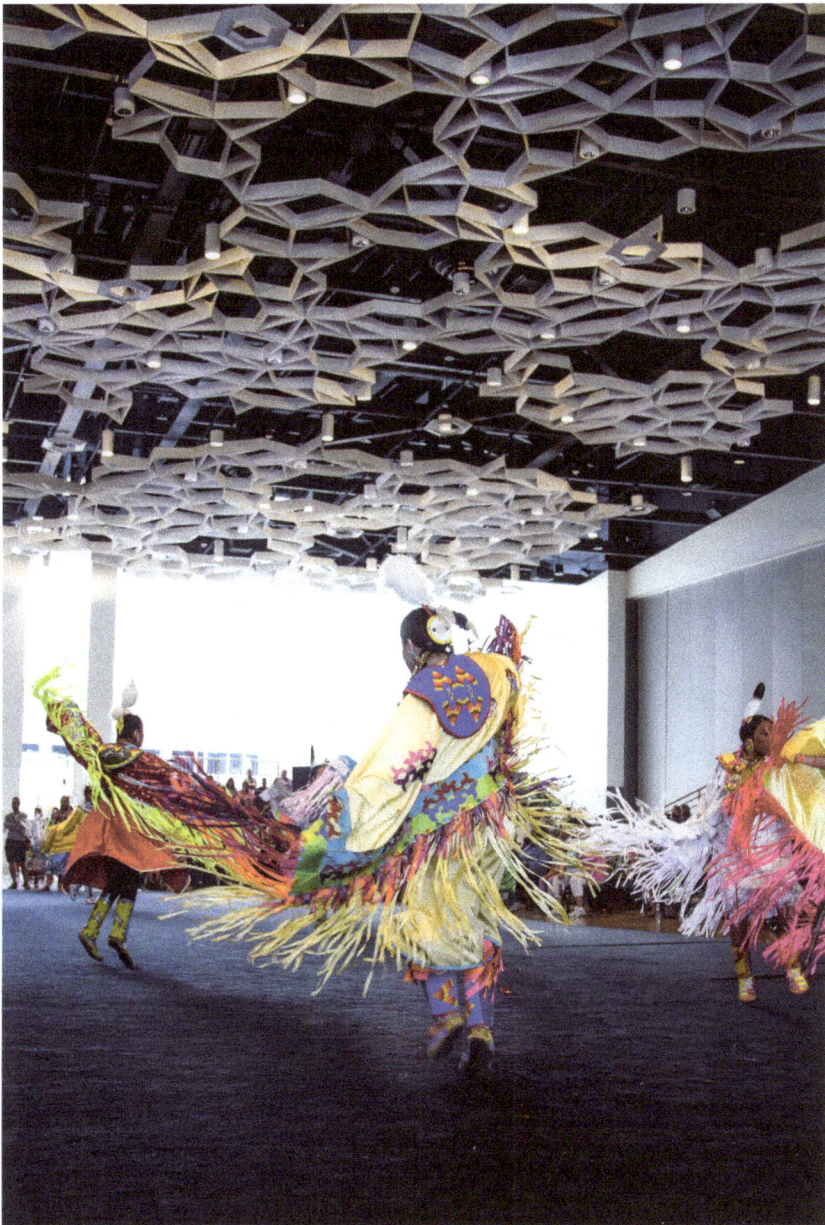

Figure 8.1 Fancy Shawl dancers performing at Manito Ahbee 2016 International Pow Wow. Photograph by Ginger Johnson.

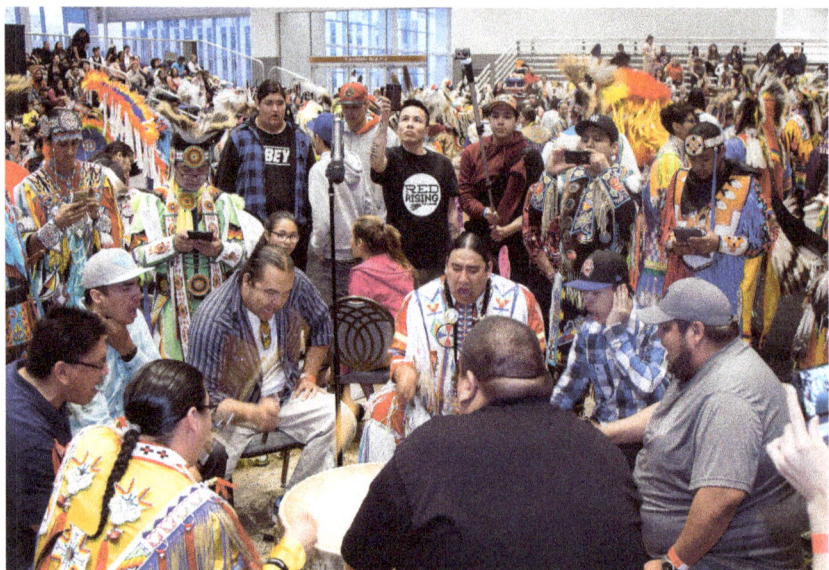

Figure 8.2 Drum group performing at Manito Ahbee 2016 International Pow Wow. Photograph by Ginger Johnson.

73; Perea 2014: 27–28), holds at most powwows: women typically do not sit at or play the drums. It is not unusual, however, for female singers to stand just outside the circle of seated drummers and sing along with them, sometimes at the same pitch and sometimes an octave higher. There do exist drum groups with female members, and indeed all-woman drum groups, but these remain in the minority.

The powwow emerged in the United States during the late nineteenth century, drawing on traditional Plains songs and dances on the one hand and influences from the Wild West show on the other (Levine 2013). It has since then spread across North America, including ones whose traditional musical and choreographic practices are very different from those of the Plains (see Powers 1990; Goertzen 2001; Browner 2002 and 2009; Hoefnagels 2002; Whidden 2007). Thus, although the contemporary powwow incorporates practices from First Nations whose traditional territories coincide with what is now Manitoba, its presence in many communities is relatively recent, and during fieldwork I talked to a number of Indigenous elders who did not witness their first powwow until well after World War Two.

Some powwows are competitive events at which dancers can win significant sums of money; others (frequently distinguished as 'traditional powwows') are non-competitive gatherings held in honour of particular people or to mark special community occasions (see Scales 2007 and 2012). While powwows are open and public when compared to more traditional ceremonies, they nevertheless incorporate a number of sacred elements (see Scales 2012: 60–61). In Manitoba they open with prayer, and sometimes a pipe ceremony; dance outfits frequently incorporate elements that reflect the dancer's spiritual characteristics; and drums are honoured through the observance of special protocols.[4]

Drum song at these events engages the senses in distinctive ways, involving hearing as well as the bodily experiences of singing and dancing to the songs. (As this suggests, although this chapter focuses on hearing, it is also concerned with the senses more broadly.) Beginning with hearing, the most immediately notable characteristic of powwow music is its volume (see Perea 2014: 16–17). Powwow drums are large, loud instruments, and their volume can be overwhelming when all of the members of a drum group are singing at the tops of their voices and striking the centre of the drum skin in unison with their drumsticks (it can be even more so when the singing is amplified, as it is at larger powwows).

Other vocal elements of powwow song are also remarkable. In the northern style of singing that predominates where I do my research, singers perform with tense voices, beginning each song at the top of their vocal register in an arresting wail (lower-pitched singing is more common in other parts of the continent). As noted, most drum groups are made up entirely of men, and the result is the sound of a chorus of male voices at their limits. A third notable element is the texture of the music: the singers perform in unison (and occasionally octaves), accompanied only by the sound of the drum and any instruments that are part of dancers' clothing: for example, the metal cones that make up part of the Jingle Dress regalia. Lastly, what is sung is also distinctive; much of it consists of vocables (sung, non-lexical syllables), for instance, 'wey-yah-hey-yah' or 'wey-hey-yo'. Words, meanwhile, tend to be in Indigenous rather than settler languages.

Does everyone – insiders and outsiders, those who grew up hearing such singing and those who did not – hear these aspects of powwow singing as 'distinctive' or 'striking'? It may be more accurate to say that to most

---

4   For instance, Scales describes how the area around a drum is kept clean at a powwow, how the drum is always left attended, and how sweetgrass may be burned for it (2012: 75, 123–24).

North American listeners, Indigenous and non-Indigenous, powwow songs sound markedly different from the songs that predominate in the settler public sphere (i.e. in public contexts in which non-Indigenous participants are in the majority). They are in a more extreme vocal register, they are sung with more vocal tension, and they have a sparser texture, involving a single melodic line supported by a drum, rather than a combination of vocal and instrumental forces that generate harmony. Further, much of the singing is wordless.

The singing also engages other senses in those who take part. Perhaps most notable for the adult male singers who make up the majority of practitioners is the experience of moving between states of vocal tension and relaxation. Songs in the northern style, as mentioned, begin at the very top of the male range, gradually descending to a much lower pitch during the course of each strophe.[5] The name given to strophes in this music – push-ups – captures this trajectory nicely. It is less indicative of the experience of female singers: women often sing in the same octave as men at the beginning of a strophe – well within a comfortable vocal range – and then shift into a higher octave when the melody moves too low. As this suggests, language about the singing tends to assume masculine experience as the default.

Northern-style singing offers a number of opportunities for the gendered performance of effortful musical labour. Male singers occasionally clutch their throats at the beginning of a push-up, constricting their larynxes to help them attain the spectacular high notes characteristic of this style of singing (see Scales 2012: 80). Singing also involves exertions that can injure singers, and it is not unusual to hear simultaneously proud and rueful statements that one's throat hurts after having sung too much over a weekend. (Some singers find strategies to achieve the desired vocal sound without strain or pain, it is important to add.)

Many of those who listen to powwow songs are dancers, of course. Indeed, dancers need to listen closely and attend to the formal structure of songs, since it is expected that, in performance, they will stop exactly on the final beat of the last strophe (in some cases, a song they are hearing for the very first time). Many of the dance styles performed at powwows are physically demanding, so hearing and attending to songs accompanies activity that is both exhausting and exhilarating.

---

5 On the structure of powwow songs, see Browner 2002 and 2009; Levine and Nettl 2011; Scales 2012.

GOSPEL SONG

In gospel singing, the second of the singing practices to be considered here, Native singers perform a mixture of hymns, songs associated with the Pentecostal tradition, and popular songs on Christian themes. These make use of European harmonic and melodic conventions and are sung to guitar, rather than drum, accompaniment, in a manner closely informed by the stylistic conventions of the popular genre of country music. All of this may seem a long way from drum songs that address spirit grandmothers and grandfathers (Anishinaabe people often refer to spirits using these terms). Yet a number of factors make it clear that gospel songs are also Indigenous music.[6] They are often sung in Aboriginal languages and at gatherings where the great majority of attendees are Native, and they are an integral component of funerary rituals that play an important part in community life (of which more shortly). Perhaps not surprisingly, a number of my research participants regularly attend both events where drum song is heard and gatherings where gospel song is performed. Some of the older ones were familiar with Christian hymns long before they heard the drum songs associated with the powwow (the dissemination by missionaries of hymns in Cree and Anishinaabe communities began in the middle of the nineteenth century, perhaps a century before modern powwow singing and dancing arrived in some places).

Gospel singing is heard in church services, but associated in an especially close way with gatherings where clergy are less visible: informal singing sessions and (especially) funerary rituals. When someone dies, the community often holds a wake for one or more nights before the funeral. Family and friends sit with the deceased, while groups and individuals take turns singing gospel songs through the night. While clergy sometimes contribute to the gathering, it is above all community members who attend to the bereaved in song. Both men and women participate in the singing, whether as soloists or choristers (although men are much more likely to occupy roles as members of the bands that accompany the singing). This way of observing the death of a loved one is common enough that the Aboriginal Funeral Chapel, a business in Winnipeg's North End, advertises itself specifically to families that wish to hold overnight services.

The songs heard at wakes are much more like the music that predominates in the mainstreams of North American public life than drum

---

6 On 'unexpected' Indigenous musics, see Perea 2012, which draws on Deloria's work on 'Indians in unexpected places' (Deloria 2004).

song: the repertoire makes use of strophic patterns and a harmonic and melodic language that can be found in musics of European origin from nineteenth-century hymns onward. All the same, this music is marked in certain ways, most notably through the use of elements borrowed from country music, including a tense vocal style and ornaments known as cry breaks – 'constrictions of the vocal articulatory mechanism that "pinch" a note in midstream, producing either momentary silence or grace-note movements into falsetto registers' (Fox 2004: 280–281). Thus, while gospel singing connects Indigenous communities to wider realms of Christian practice, it does so through sounds associated with rural and working-class musical life.

Notable in the experience of performing this music is a sense of physical negotiation. Many gospel songs follow straightforward formulas and can be accompanied using just a few guitar chords. This makes the music amenable to not only participation by non-specialists, but also impromptu performances between people who do not regularly make music together. Wakes frequently bring together musicians from different communities and congregations (see Dueck 2013: 109), so such spur-of-the-moment collaborations are not uncommon. However, different singers frequently perform the same songs in ways that are rhythmically distinctive, sometimes idiosyncratically so, and their collaborators are often forced to make rapid recalibrations to accommodate unexpected musical shifts.

The wakes at which gospel music is sung are notable for not only their inclusivity but their length, and their demands on participants. As noted, singing starts in the evening and often goes on until early in the morning, and it is not unusual for a wake to run for two or even three nights. Singers can travel long distances to take part in these events, then stay up late once they arrive. So, while the most obvious sensory component of the wake is the sound of song, physical fatigue is also a factor, experienced to various degrees by participants depending on their roles.

Musicians understand singing at the wake as an act of comfort. Singer Emery Marsden told me:

> When I started going to wakes ... the first thing that I heard was 'Amazing Grace' and 'In the Sweet By and By' and all these songs. ... I used to see people get uplifted by these songs, and they'd sit there all night and sing these psalms and comfort the family that would be mourning. But I'd sit there at times myself ... there's times when my loved ones passed away ... I used to sit there and I'd listen to the people that would sing .... It would be like having a cup of coffee. I'd sit there and I'd listen, and the mourning part of me would

be at ease because of the music. (Interview with the author, August 2003, quoted in Dueck 2013: 111)

Marsden's words, even now, evoke for me very specific memories: nights spent surrounded by gospel singing; singers arriving at a wake with cups of takeout coffee in hand; a table of food and drink, a large percolator in the middle, at a late-night vigil at the Aboriginal Funeral Chapel.

Through his everyday simile, Marsden invited me to think of song as a substance that acts on its recipients. In the same way that a cup of coffee warms hands and stomach, music consoles the bereaved (see Dueck 2013: 111–112). The singer's image imparted rhetorical weight to his claim concerning the efficacy of music, rendering song as warming, infilling stuff, something more than mere sound.

MUSIC AND THE SACRED SENSORIUM

Marsden's image of song as a substance may seem unremarkable, but it invites reflection for exactly this reason – and here I move beyond my interview with him to consider why it seems appropriate to speak of music in similar ways in many different cultural contexts. It probably has to do in part with the way that sound is conveyed through substances, especially fluid media such as the air. It also has to do with the sense that one can be immersed in or *surrounded* by sound in the same way one might be by air, smoke or water.[7] Further, many kinds of music are sustained and *ongoing* (consider how Marsden speaks of coffee, a substance that one imbibes over time, that warms drinkers, that keeps them awake). This ongoing-ness is true of both the traditional sacred song and Christian music described earlier, in which the sustained sounds of voices are accompanied by more rapidly decaying but nonetheless regular noises: of drums and rattles in traditional music and of the guitar in gospel singing. It is also true of many musics beyond those considered in this chapter – although the concepts of fluidness and ongoing-ness seem particularly appropriate when one reflects on the sensation of singing, in which one feels oneself producing sustained sound as one controls how one's breath exits the body.

---

7 There is a resonance here with a remark in McLuhan and Fiore's *The Medium is the Massage*: 'We are *enveloped* by sound. It forms a seamless web around us. We say, "Music shall fill the air." We never say, "Music shall fill a particular segment of the air"' (1967: 111; emphasis in original).

Sound is treated as substance in sacred contexts far from those that are the focus of this chapter. Consider for example the following description of 'spells accompanied by simple rites of impregnation' from Malinowksi's discussion of the magic practices of Trobriand Islanders in *Argonauts of the Western Pacific*:

> In [a number of performances of spells of impregnation] an object is put well within reach of the voice, and in an appropriate position. Often, the object is placed within a receptacle or covering so that the voice enters an enclosed space and is concentrated upon the substance to be charged. ... [For example], the adze blade is first of all half wrapped up in a banana leaf, and the voice enters the blade and the inside of the leaf, which subsequently is folded over and tied over the blade. (1932 [1922]: 405)

In Malinowski's description, the words and sounds of the charm are not only concentrated on their object, as substances whose flow is directed, but physically wrapped in place around it.[8]

In many other contexts as well, talk and behaviour highlight the substantial aspect of sacred sound. Why is this? One answer is that sound, perhaps especially musical sound, is amenable, by means of a vague and mutable iconicity, to the representation of otherwise invisible processes and persons. I draw the term 'iconicity' from the semiotics of Charles Sanders Peirce, who describes an icon as a symbol that represents its referent by means of some similarity of form.[9] The relationship between the sound in a stethoscope and the beating of an unseen heart is one example; the relationship between the increasing volume of a voice and the growing closeness of the speaker is another. I argue that sound is well-suited to representing sacred processes and presences by a similar kind of iconic signification (although people and groups make use of this affordance in a range of ways, some more established or sanctioned than others).

To elaborate, sacred sounds lend themselves in the first place to accomplishing things: enacting invisible or abstract *processes*. In the Indigenous communities where I do research, surrounding a bereaved community member with song extends comfort, while singing an honour song to a person or spirit being communicates reverence. Another example is the process of invocation: music is often bound up with the summoning of

---

8 This observation was inspired by remarks by Michael Silverstein in one of his 2002 'Language in Culture' lectures at the University of Chicago.

9 See Peirce (1960: 143); on iconicity as it relates especially to music, see Turino (1999: 226–27, 242–44; 2008: 6–8).

spirit beings. At many formal Indigenous assemblies, it is common to sing songs that invite specific spirits to come into the presence of those who have gathered. Other examples can be found in musics of possession: the music at the Shona *bira* summons ancestors (see Berliner 1993 [1978]: 186–206), and the melodies of Tunisian *stambēlī* 'coax [spirits] to descend into the bodies of dancing hosts' (Jankowsky 2010: 2). Further, music may enact more than one process simultaneously: many Christians understand congregational singing not only to convey praise to God, but also to transmit God's blessings back to worshippers. Melvin Butler writes, 'Music in the Pentecostal church is a vehicle for praising and worshiping God and in return receiving the spiritual strength to persevere through life's hardships. In the words of a well-known gospel chorus, "When praises go up, blessings come down"' (Butler 2000: 33).

Sacred music also lends itself to representing the *presence* of beings or powers. This is most evident in instances when it evokes or triggers states that correspond to what one might feel in those presences: exhilaration, awe, a transformation of the experience of passing time. Sacred presences may also be associated with sounds within the music. In the singing of Sardinian confraternities described by Bernard Lortat-Jacob, four-man choirs sing devotional music in harmony in a way that can produce the *quintina*, an apparent fifth voice associated with the Virgin Mary (1998: 15, 151–152).[10] Lortat-Jacob writes:

> the *quintina* is a woman: the gender of the word attests it, but more still the timbre, light and ethereal, contrasting with that of the powerful male voices that produce it. The *Miserere*, the *Jesu*, or the *Stabba* [pieces sung by the groups] therefore take on the aspect of a long lamentation that the dramatic context of the Passion invites hearing as that of the Virgin. (1998: 152, translation by the present author)

Sensory practices other than music similarly lend themselves to the representation of the unseen through their surrounding-ness, indwelling-ness and ongoing-ness. Indigenous ceremonial practice alone contains many examples. At a range of gatherings, smudging (censing) with burning sage effects the purification of persons and objects. Certain ceremonies involve the voluntary endurance of hunger or pain, by which participants earn the pity of the Great Spirit. And in the sweat lodge (a ceremony in

---

10 This is an effect of certain harmonics being reinforced when the singers blend their voices in a particular way. See also Bithell (1999: 118).

which participants sit in a domed hut around heated stones over which water is poured) those taking part are surrounded by heat and steam at the same time that they are in the presence of spirits. Yet other sustained and immersive sensory experiences are encountered in the chapters in this volume; see for example Anne Katrine de Hemmer Gudme's discussion of the smells of sacred observance.

To sum up the argument so far, participants in ritual represent sacred presences and processes by means of iconic sensory experiences that they themselves generate; music, thanks to its surrounding-ness, infilling-ness and ongoing-ness, lends itself particularly well to this. The argument has some formal similarities to Durkheim's theory that social groups misinterpret their social power as a sacred force originating outside themselves (Durkheim 1995 [1912]). There is an important difference, however: the theory advanced here does not require naive participants to misunderstand music – or the transformations engendered by hearing, producing or moving to it – as the represented process or presence itself. Music may embody the presence/process or merely symbolise or accompany it, and participants may or may not be 'naive'.

A few more general caveats can also be noted. First, not all religious practices make use of music's mutable potential for iconicity, and not all uses of this potential are religious.[11] For example, music is regarded with suspicion or ambivalence in a number of manifestations of both Christianity and Islam. Second, although the iconicity of these surrounding, ongoing and indwelling sensations is often compelling, it does not determine reactions. It rather affords a range of responses and interpretations, collective and personal, official and demotic. This is evident in research done by Owen Coggins on drone metal (2016), a genre of popular music whose canonical recordings feature long, low, heavily distorted sonorities, and in which religious imagery and even quotations from religious texts appear. Drone metal epitomises the capacity of music to engage the senses in immersive ways, particularly in live performances where it is heard at deafeningly loud volume. But the interviews Coggins conducted with listeners indicate they have no difficulty distinguishing immersive sensory experiences from experiences they understand as religious, even when there might be good reasons for them to blur the categories. Coggins writes, 'For listeners who [stated] commitment to particular religions, aspects of drone metal

---

11   The idea of a potential that actors may or may not activate resonates with the concept of musical affordances described by writers such as Tia DeNora (2000: 39–40) and Martin Clayton (2001: 6–9).

described as ritual and even spiritual or mystical were generally compared with, but sharply differentiated from, each [listener's] religious practice' (2016: 254).

All the same, immersive and indwelling experiences are widely associated with spiritual processes and presences, and music seems to afford particularly significant opportunities for this by means of an iconicity that can stand for many things. Consider again the drums used in Indigenous song, which are at once incorporated in songs that summon spirits and understood to have spirits themselves. Their sound is both a signal used as part of the *process* of invoking spirits and a sign of the *presence* of the spirit of the drum. This flexible iconicity is probably one reason why, across many times and places, there has been a close connection between religion on the one hand and music, song and heightened speech on the other.[12]

MUSIC'S PLACE IN THE INDIGENOUS SACRED SENSORIUM

Having outlined a general argument concerning music and the sacred sensorium, I return here to the specificities of the music-making with which I began. How do these singing practices distinguish an *Indigenous* sensorium?

They do so in part through the markedness of particular vocal sounds. The high, tense sound of northern-style drum singing is one of the definitive sonic indices of North American Indigeneity, for insiders and outsiders alike. In contrast, the vocal sound of country gospel music has much wider associations, namely with working-class and rural audiences where non-Indigenous people are in the majority. Yet these vocal sounds, too, instantiate distinctiveness, given that many Native people share a working-class habitus and ties to rural communities. And, while powwow song affirms a legacy of Indigenous musical practice, it has more in common with gospel singing than might initially be apparent: both reflect a history of colonialism.[13] Returning to the main point, while the music that helps to

---

12 Bruno Nettl, in a core ethnomusicological text, suggests that one of the primary purposes of music across cultures is to 'control humanity's relationship to the supernatural, mediating between human and other beings' (2005: 253).

13 A great deal of contemporary drum song makes use of musical structures closely related to the powwow, which, as noted earlier, has roots in part in early Wild West shows. The 'country' vocal style associated with gospel music, meanwhile, is closely associated with romantic images of a frontier West. In short, both singing styles stand in dialogue with realms of commercial culture

distinguish spaces of Indigenous sacred observance is not always unique to Indigenous people, it nevertheless differentiates those spaces: from settler society in the case of drum song, and from middle-class music worlds in the case of gospel singing.[14]

Indigenous musical and sacred life are also distinguished by their approaches to temporality and participation. Ceremonies, rites of passage and social gatherings often last for long spans of time: some traditional ceremonies are held over the course of four days; wakes run through the night, and sometimes for more than one night. These events feature nearly constant music-making by a series of musicians and/or groups. Important events tend to take up time, articulated through a steady succession of singers and songs (cf. Nettl 2001: 259). They also allow for extensive musical participation, being guided by the principle that anyone who wishes should be able to take part, specialists and non-specialists alike. Ceremonies, rites of passage and social gatherings thus present opportunities for multiple participants to make contributions that express their particularity within a context of collective endeavour.

Perhaps paradoxically, the inclusiveness of events at which gospel song is performed allows for individuality to be highlighted. As noted earlier, it is not unusual for gospel singers to have highly distinctive takes on familiar pieces. When such musicians come together to perform, as often happens at wakes, their individual approaches often necessitate mid-performance scrambles to accommodate unexpected musical turns, interactions that instantiate personal idiosyncrasy with especial immediacy. The experience of making music in these circumstances is both a moment of collaboration and an embodied encounter with unruly personal difference.

Other than the fact that it is Indigenous people who are involved, how are the inclusive, participatory and particularity-friendly spaces discussed here – and the kinds of sensations cultivated in them – Indigenous? This question seems especially pertinent given that gospel singing is not a strictly Indigenous musical activity (see Quick 2016). I suggest that drum song and wake singing continue an emphasis, evident in older Northern Algonquian sacred practice, on the importance of particular individuals and their gifts to their communities. In the Ojibwe and Cree hunting

---

that have mediated colonial understandings of Indigeneity (which is not to say that they repeat these understandings in any straightforward way; see Dueck 2013: 25–26, 73–81).

14 I borrow the term 'music worlds' from Ruth Finnegan (2007 [1989]) who in turn bases it on Howard Becker's concept of 'art worlds' (Becker 2008 [1982]).

communities studied in the middle of the twentieth century by anthropologists such as A. I. Hallowell (1955 and 1992), Leonard Mason (1967) and Edward Rogers (1962), the most central sacred experiences traditionally took the form of encounters with spirits dreamed in the course of a solitary fast. It was similarly through dreams that new sacred ceremonies and their attendant songs, dances and regalia were gifted to particular persons (see Landes 1968). In these ways, religious experience was highly individuated. At the same time, those blessed through dream encounters employed their gifts for the good of their communities. Contemporary forms of Indigenous assembly – in which long spans of time allow for contributions from both specialists and non-specialists, and in which individual idiosyncrasy both enriches and complicates collective action – enact a form of continuity with these older aspects of Northern Algonquian sacred life.[15]

CONCLUSION

In this chapter I have considered two forms of sacred music practised in Indigenous communities in and around the western Canadian city of Winnipeg: drum song and gospel singing. Reflection on these led in the first place to the idea that the surrounding-ness, infilling-ness and ongoingness of music lend themselves to the mediation of sacred presences and processes. Such mediations, though hardly universal, are widespread, and music, by means of its potential for iconicity, seems particularly suited to them. Reflection on the two singing practices secondly suggested how it is that Native communities in this part of North America cultivate an Indigenous sacred sensorium. They do so by using distinctive vocal styles, by holding gatherings that are participatory and temporally expansive, and by undertaking forms of music-making that foreground both the challenges and benefits of inclusion. In exploring the two singing practices, I did not seek to distinguish the degree to which their musical components represent an authentic Indigeneity. I characterised both as Indigenous, not out of any particular sympathy for Christianity, or in an attempt to deny the devastating impact of colonialism on Aboriginal religion, but rather in acknowledgement that both are widely practised in Indigenous communities and that both lend themselves to the elaboration of certain valued modes of Northern Algonquian sociability.

15 I make this case at greater length in Dueck (2013).

It remains to draw together the general and the specific arguments. Music's mutable iconicity presents general opportunities for representing sacred presences and processes, but these are realised in culturally specific ways. It is important to the communities discussed in this chapter that their members should pass long nights comforting the bereaved, and that these times together should allow anyone who has something to contribute to participate. It matters that the sound of adult male voices at their limits should be a privileged part of drum songs, and that these songs should be sung as a mixture of vocables and words in Indigenous languages. That the gendered division of labour in drum song is subject to contemporary negotiation indicates that how music is deployed changes over time, but this does not alter a more fundamental point: that communities make use of music's affordances for sacred experience in highly particularised ways.

REFERENCES

Becker, H. S. 2008 [1982]. *Art Worlds: 25th Anniversary Edition: Updated and Expanded.* Berkeley: University of California Press.

Berliner, P. 1993 [1978]. *The Soul of Mbira: Music and Traditions of the Shona People of Zimbabwe.* Chicago: The University of Chicago Press.

Bithell, C. 1999. 'Review-essay on Lortat-Jacob, B., *Chants de Passion*', *British Journal of Ethnomusicology* 8: 116–122. https://doi.org/10.1080/09681229908567284

Browner, T. 2002. *Heartbeat of the People: Music and Dance of the Northern Pow-wow.* Urbana: University of Illinois Press.

Browner, T. 2009. 'An Acoustical Geography of Intertribal Pow-wow Songs' in T. Browner (ed.), *Music of the First Nations: Tradition and Innovation in Native North America.* Urbana: University of Illinois Press. pp. 131–140.

Bucko, R. A. 1998. *The Lakota Ritual of the Sweat Lodge: History and Contemporary Practice.* Lincoln: University of Nebraska Press.

Butler, M. L. 2000. 'Musical Style and Experience in a Brooklyn Pentecostal Church: An "Insider's" Perspective', *Current Musicology* 70: 33–60.

Clayton, M. 2001. 'Introduction: Towards a Theory of Musical Meaning (In India and Elsewhere)', *British Journal of Ethnomusicology* 10.1: 1–17. https://doi.org/10.1080/09681220108567307

Coggins, O. 2016. *Drone Metal Mysticism*, PhD thesis, Faculty of Arts, The Open University.

Deloria, E. 1929. 'The Sun Dance of the Oglala Sioux', *The Journal of American Folklore* 42.166: 354–413. https://doi.org/10.2307/535232

Deloria, P. J. 2004. *Indians in Unexpected Places.* Lawrence: University Press of Kansas.

DeNora, T. 2000. *Music in Everyday Life.* Cambridge, Cambridge University Press. https://doi.org/10.1017/CBO9780511489433

Diamond, B., Cronk, M.S., and von Rosen, F. 1994. *Visions of Sound: Musical Instruments of First Nations Communities in Northeastern America.* Chicago: The University of Chicago Press.

Dueck, B. 2013. *Musical Intimacies and Indigenous Imaginaries: Aboriginal Music and Dance in Public Performance*. New York: Oxford University Press. https://doi.org/10.1093/acprof:oso/9780199747641.001.0001

Durkheim, E. 1995 [1912]. *The Elementary Forms of Religious Life*. New York: The Free Press.

Ellis, C., Lassiter, L.E., and Dunham, G.H. (eds). 2005. *Powwow*. Lincoln: University of Nebraska Press.

Finnegan, R. 2007 [1989]. *The Hidden Musicians: Music-Making in an English Town* (2nd edn). Middletown, CT: Wesleyan University Press.

Fox, A. A. 2004. *Real Country: Music and Language in Working-Class Culture*. Durham: Duke University Press. https://doi.org/10.1215/9780822385998

Goertzen, C. 2001. 'Powwows and Identity on the Piedmont and Coastal Plains of North Carolina', *Ethnomusicology* 45.1: 58–88. https://doi.org/10.2307/852634

Hallowell, A. I. 1955. *Culture and Experience*. Philadelphia: Pennsylvania University Press. https://doi.org/10.9783/9781512816600

Hallowell, A. I. 1992. *The Ojibwa of Berens River: Ethnography into History*, edited with a preface and afterword by J. S. H. Brown. Fort Worth, TX: Harcourt Brace Jovanovich College Publishers.

Hoefnagels, A. 2002. 'Powwow Songs: Travelling Songs and Changing Protocol', *World of Music* 44.1: 127–36.

Jankowsky, R. C. 2010. *Stambeli: Music, Trance, and Alterity in Tunisia*. Chicago: The University of Chicago Press. https://doi.org/10.7208/chicago/9780226392202.001.0001

Landes, R. 1968. *Ojibwa Religion and the Midéwiwin*. Madison: University of Wisconsin Press.

Levine, V. L. 2013. 'Powwow', *Grove Music Online, Oxford Music Online*, http://www.oxfordmusiconline.com.libezproxy.open.ac.uk/subscriber/article/grove/music/A2252169 (consulted 1 August 2016).

Levine, V. L. and Nettl, B. 2011. 'Strophic Form and Asymmetrical Repetition in Four American Indian Songs' in M. Tenzer and J. Roeder, J. (eds), *Analytical and Cross-Cultural Studies in World Music*. New York: Oxford University Press. pp. 288–315. https://doi.org/10.1093/acprof:oso/9780195384581.003.0008

Lortat-Jacob, B. 1998. *Chants de passion: Au coeur d'une confrérie de Sardaigne*. Paris: Les Éditions du Cerf.

Malinowski, B. 1932 [1922]. *Argonauts of the Western Pacific: An Account of Native Enterprise and Adventure in the Archipelagoes of Melanesian New Guinea* (2nd impression). London: Routledge.

Mason, L. 1967. *The Swampy Cree: A Study in Acculturation*. Ottawa: National Museum of Canada, Department of the Secretary of State.

McLuhan, M., and Fiore, Q. 1967. *The Medium Is the Massage: An Inventory of Effects*. New York: Bantam Books.

Nettl, B. 2001. 'Native American Music' in B. Nettl, C. Capwell, P. V. Bohlman, I. K. F. Wong and T. Turino, *Excursions in World Music* (3rd edn). Upper Saddle River, NJ: Prentice Hall. pp. 255–273.

Nettl, B. 2005. *The Study of Ethnomusicology: Thirty-one Issues and Concepts* (2nd edition). Urbana: University of Illinois Press.

Peirce, C. S. 1960. *Collected Papers*, Vols. 1 and 2: *Principles of Philosophy* and *Elements of Logic*, edited by C. Hartshorne and P. Weiss. Cambridge, MA: Belknap Press of Harvard University Press.

Perea, J.-C. 2012. 'The Unexpectedness of Jim Pepper', *MUSICultures* 39.1: 70–82.

Perea, J-C. 2014. *Intertribal Native American Music in the United States: Experiencing Music, Expressing Culture*. New York: Oxford University Press.

Powers, W. K. 1990. *War Dance: Plains Indian Musical Performance*. Tucson: University of Arizona Press.

Quick, S. 2016. 'Review, *Musical Intimacies and Indigenous Imaginaries: Aboriginal Music and Dance in Public Performance* by B. Dueck', *Ethnomusicology* 60.1: 178–181. https://doi.org/10.5406/ethnomusicology.60.1.0178

Rogers, E. S. 1962. *The Round Lake Ojibwa*. Toronto: Art and Archaeology Division, Royal Ontario Museum, University of Toronto.

Scales, C. A. 2007. 'Powwows, Intertribalism, and the Value of Competition', *Ethnomusicology* 51.1: 1–29.

Scales, C. A. 2012. *Recording Culture: Powwow Music and the Aboriginal Recording Industry on the Northern Plains*. Durham: Duke University Press.
https://doi.org/10.1215/9780822395720

Turino, T. 1999. 'Signs of Imagination, Identity, and Experience: A Peircian Semiotic Theory for Music', *Ethnomusicology* 43.2: 221–255. https://doi.org/10.2307/852734

Turino, T. 2008. *Music as Social Life: The Politics of Participation*. Chicago: The University of Chicago Press.

Whidden, L. 2007. *Essential Song: Three Decades of Northern Cree Music*. Waterloo, ON: Wilfrid Laurier University Press.

Byron Dueck is Senior Lecturer and Head of Music at The Open University, UK. He is the author of *Musical Intimacies and Indigenous Imaginaries: Aboriginal Music in Public Performance* (Oxford University Press, 2013), and co-editor, with Martin Clayton and Laura Leante, of *Experience and Meaning in Musical Performance* (Oxford University Press, 2013).

Section Five
TOUCH

Chapter 9

The Texture of the Gift: Religious Touching in the Greco-Roman World

JESSICA HUGHES

What did ancient religion feel like? This chapter contemplates the tactile profile of Greco-Roman religion by revisiting a selection of objects and practices from ancient Mediterranean contexts. The sense of touch permeated any visit to a classical temple. Some tactile experiences were shared by nearly everyone who entered the sanctuary, like the casual skin-to-stone contact with the monumental architecture, or the washing of hands in the water of purificatory basins. Other types of contact would have been restricted to certain cult officials, such as the unpacking of the sticky animal organs used in divination, or the cleansing and anointing of fragile ancient cult images made from wood or ivory. In Greco-Roman art, touch is often used as a powerful visual symbol of contact with the divine: vase paintings and reliefs show mortals clasping cult statues in desperate acts of supplication (Figure 9.1), while healing deities in sculpted reliefs lay hands on the bodies of their ailing supplicants (see Figure 9.2). And although artistic scenes like these cannot be taken as documentary evidence for actual tactile experiences, they can nevertheless help us to understand some of the complex, culturally-specific ways in which touch was given meaning by ancient worshippers.

This chapter begins with a general introduction to some of the most common tactile stimuli encountered in sanctuaries across the Greco-Roman world. I focus in particular on ritual cleansing, votives and divine healing, since these things are particularly relevant for the discussion that follows. After this, I move on to my main case study of the so-called 'confession stelai' – a group of inscribed stone tablets which were dedicated

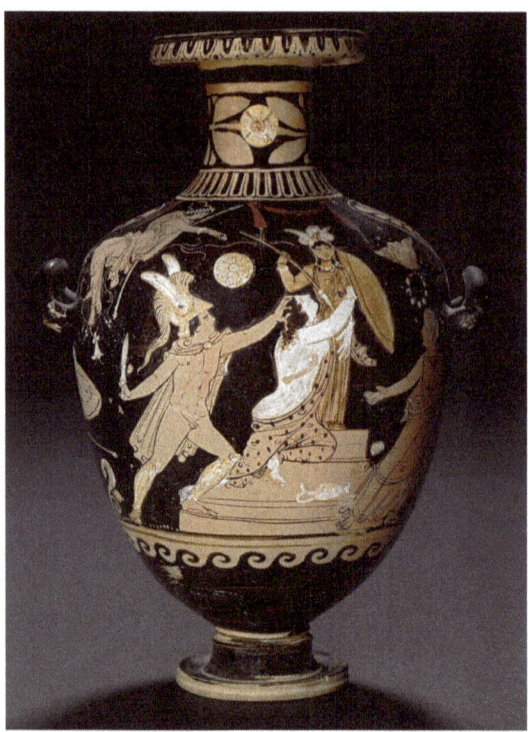

Figure 9.1 Red-figured South Italian hydria showing the assault of the priestess Cassandra by the Lesser Ajax in the temple of Athena at Troy, 340–320 BCE. Height 33 cm. British Museum 1824,0501.35. © The Trustees of the British Museum.

between the first and third centuries CE in the rural sanctuaries of Roman Asia Minor, an area which corresponds to parts of modern Turkey. These stelai (singular *stele* or *stela*) record a series of ritual transgressions committed by local people who had been punished by the gods, and who were thus erecting the stone tablets as part of a process of reparation and forgiveness. As we shall see, the sense of touch plays a central role in these inscriptions and the intimate stories that they recount. My discussion here identifies three main tactile themes: first, the transgressive touching of forbidden objects and bodies by mortals; second, the punitive touching of the mortal body by the gods; and finally the asynchronous touching of religious objects in the sanctuary by both mortal and divine hands. This last theme has a much wider relevance for how we understand the role of material artefacts that were left in Greco-Roman sanctuaries, which were designed not only to capture the attention of the gods who lived there, but also to encourage their tactile engagement.

ENTERING THE CLASSICAL SANCTUARY

A tourist pulls up in the car park of an archaeological site in Sicily. She climbs out of the car, stretching her legs after the long journey, and lifts her toddler daughter out of the booster-seat in the back. Slamming the car door shut, they walk slowly over to the ticket office, stopping momentarily to buy a bottle of water from the vendor parked outside the gates. Clutching bottle, map and tickets, the woman lifts her daughter into her arms. It's only April, but already hot. Once inside the barrier of the site, they move into the shade of an almond tree, and sit down on the spiky, uncomfortable earth. The woman squints at the already-crumpled paper map, then looks across to the huge stone temples that stand along the Via Sacra. How different they appear from in the photographs! Far in the distance, she sees people are climbing on the temple steps and base, periodically vanishing between the enormous marble columns. The woman takes a flower from her daughter's hand, and absent-mindedly brushes it against her lips. Then, standing up again, she gathers up her camera, water, map and bag, hoists her daughter onto her hip, and starts to walk slowly towards the temples.

In the modern tourist experience of ancient sites, the sense of touch looms large. Certain textures are new and unfamiliar, the air feels hotter (or colder) than that of our habitual environments, and we are often preoccupied with feeling around for the assortment of accessories that we bring with us on our journey – cameras, phones, guidebooks, snacks, hotel and car keys, and so on. Our movement around the sites is carefully choreographed ('No Entry', 'Exit This Way'), and physical contact with objects or buildings is often frowned upon or explicitly forbidden ('Please Do Not Touch the Wall-Paintings'). These prohibitions often simply accentuate our desire to reach out and touch the fabric of the ancient buildings we pass through – a desire born from curiosity about different materials, but also from the frisson of delight at the possibility that *we might touch what they touched*. Materials like marble, we know, existed right at the beginning of a temple's life, therefore they seem to offer us the quasi-magical capacity to dissolve boundaries between past and present, and even to disavow the ephemerality of the human body (i.e. by bringing ancient 'hands' back to life). Peter Dent has recently explored these issues in relation to a marble column in the cathedral at Santiago de Compostela, in which a handprint has been eroded into the marble by hundreds of generations of touching pilgrims. 'Looking at the handprint', he writes, 'is like tracing the weight and motion of bodies worn into old flagstones, the passage of many feet that mark out paths of action and acceptable gestures for those who follow after' (Dent 2014: 4).

What about the ancient Greco-Roman visitors? As this chapter aims to demonstrate, in classical antiquity the sense of touch was an equally salient aspect of any sanctuary visit. The range of tactile stimuli on offer, however, would have been very different, as would the meanings that these stimuli were attributed. Construction materials like marble might not have appeared quite so dominant in the landscape of the ancient sanctuary, given the wide horizon of other sculptural materials and fabrics that were originally present at these sites. In turn, although ancient sanctuaries *were* powerful sites of cultural memory (Shaya 2005), the strong symbolic function that marble has today – that is, as a 'connecting device' between past and present – was presumably not quite so central to ancient worshippers as it is for modern tourists. The marble we see today is normally pale, unlike in classical antiquity, when much of the architecture was painted and gilded. Moreover, it is fragmentary rather than whole, and physically bare rather than covered with offerings and the movable apparatus of cult. Table 9.1 lists some examples of tactile stimuli that were present in many ancient sanctuaries, together with their materials, and most common locations. The objects, bodies and rituals mentioned in this table represent only a tiny sample of things found in ancient sanctuaries; however, even this selective list can help us to appreciate the sheer variety of stimuli that might be encountered in sacred contexts, and can hint at some of the different 'modes' of touching – as in the case of the musical instruments, which were blown, hit, plucked, twanged, shaken, rattled, and so on.

On entering the sanctuary, one of the first touch-related practices that most visitors participated in was purificatory washing. This was one of the most widespread ritual activities in the Greco-Roman world. From at least the seventh century BCE, sanctuaries all over the Greco-Roman world featured washing vessels called *perirrhanteria* – wide, shallow basins made of marble, bronze or ceramic, which were placed on top of a column at approximately hand-height (Parker 1983: 20, 226–227; Paoletti 2005). These vessels were located at the entrances to sanctuaries and temples, where they engaged the sense of touch as a means of demarcating the boundary between sacred and secular territory (in this sense, they may have been the models for the holy water stoups placed at the entrance of later Christian churches). In addition to the material remains of basins, we have visual images of worshippers washing (see Ginouvès 1962 with further entries in Paoletti 2005). We also have many textual references which help to explain the significance of this act, such as the following

Table 9.1 Examples of tactile stimuli sometimes found in Greco-Roman sanctuaries

Stimulus	Material	Principal locations
The *temenos* (wall around sanctuary)	Stone	Around the periphery of the sacred space
Purificatory basins	Mainly marble, sometimes metal or ceramic, and filled with water	Often at the entrance to the sanctuary; also outside temples and by altars
Living and dead animal bodies (and excrement)	Hair/fur, flesh, blood, urine, faeces	Moving through sanctuary; eventually near altars (see Kamash, this volume)
Sacrificial implements (knives, axes, hammers)	Stone, wood, metal	Storerooms, altars
Musical instruments (includes string, wind and percussion instruments)	Wood, bronze, ivory, bone, shell, skin, alabaster	Moving towards and through sanctuary (see Petridou, this volume)
Votive offerings	Bronze, marble, terracotta, wood, hair, fabric, organic plant materials, wax, amber, limestone	Often placed around the cult statue, around altar bases
Curse tablets, binding spells and charms	Lead, papyrus, wax, broken pottery sherds, mud, hair	Wells, springs
Cult statues	Wood, marble, terracotta, ivory and gold; also fabric, leaves, branches	Often within the *naos* (inner room) of the ancient temple

passage from the late fifth-century BCE author of the Hippocratic text *On the Sacred Disease*. (Note that this passage occurs in the context of a diatribe against those physicians who attributed illness to divine causes: here, the Hippocratic author is explaining that the gods *purify* the body rather than *pollute* it.)

> We mark out the boundaries of the sanctuaries and precincts of the gods so that no one crosses them unless pure, and when we do enter, we sprinkle all around [*perirrhainesthai*] ourselves, not because we are actually in a state of being polluted, but because, if we have any possible prior taint, we might purify ourselves of it. (*On the Sacred Disease* 1.110–112)

Water, this Hippocratic author explains, was used to rid the body of invisible pollution, whether or not this had been consciously acquired. The verb *perirrhainesthai* in the passage denotes a sprinkling around the body, which was generally performed by dipping the hands (or in some instances an olive branch) into the basin, and then flicking the water droplets around the body. As Susan Guettel Cole has written, this symbolic action 'would have defined a temporal boundary around a piece of personal sacred space, creating an invisible envelope that separated the worshipper from even the incidental defilements of ordinary life' (Cole 2004: 46). Significantly for us, the discourse on pollution was also persistently tactile: not only was pollution thought to be incurred via contact with external stimuli like corpses, menstrual blood and sexualized bodies, but it is also clear from the sources that anyone who was in a state of pollution was forbidden from *touching* sacred objects. Euripides' Iphigenia, in her role as priestess of Artemis, warns of how 'if anyone touches [note that the verb used is *haptomai*] murder, or childbirth, too, or puts a hand on a corpse, believing him defiled, she [Artemis] keeps him from her altars' (Euripides *Iphigenia in Tauris* 381–383). Meanwhile, an inscribed sacred law from Philadelphia in Asia Minor obliged worshippers to demonstrate their purity by taking an oath whilst *touching the inscription* with their hands (Sokolowski 1955: no. 20; Chaniotis 2006: 139 n. 118). It is probably not surprising, then, that the method for purifying the body was also a tactual process, which involved the direct contact of the water on the skin of the immersed hands, or the sensation of sprinkled water droplets landing on the clothes and skin.

VOTIVES

Once inside the sanctuary, the range and variety of stimuli multiplied, with the individual's unique tactual experience of the visit being shaped by factors like the season, the weather, the time of day, their age, gender, disabilities and (perhaps most significantly of all) whether or not they were suffering from pain and illness. Many visitors would have brought votive offerings with them to dedicate somewhere in the sanctuary. As in later periods, votive objects in classical antiquity were used both to request help from a god, as well as to give thanks for a miracle that had already been received (often with the aim of securing the continued help and protection of the deity). Votives could be dedicated in virtually any situation, although the most common scenarios seem to have been illness and healing, fertility and procreation, as well as 'rites of passage' like the entry to adulthood or retirement from work. In turn, almost any type of object could be dedicated, so we have tens of thousands of surviving 'purpose-made' votives like figurines and models of human and animal body parts (Draycott and

Graham 2017; Hughes 2017a), but we also have traces of more personal votives that had been 'repurposed' from other areas of life – items like jewellery, toys, clothes, utensils and even hair (see Hughes 2017b for discussion of the conceptual differences between these 'purpose-made' and 're-purposed' offerings).

Votive offerings were extremely tactile objects, which were normally small enough to be carried, held and caressed by the hands of the people who offered them (and, as I shall argue below, by those who received them). The distinctive textures and materials of these objects were often inseparable from their affective, emotional qualities (Graham, forthcoming). The sensation of a frayed silk hair ribbon twisted between the fingers, the weight of a smooth amber pendant rubbing in a sweaty palm, the feel of porous terracotta under the fingernails – each of these textures and modes of touching was fundamental to how the devotee experienced the act of giving, and in turn, how the votive was 'infused' or 'contaged' with the dedicant's presence prior to dedication (a process which Amy Whitehead discusses in the next chapter of this volume). The craft materials also had an impact beyond their immediate physical, sensory qualities. People in antiquity *knew* about the processes of making – about how clay was kneaded and cooked, how bronze ore was melted, poured and moulded, how marble objects were sometimes cradled in a sculptor's lap whilst being worked with a chisel. This knowledge of sculptural process greatly expanded the range of symbolic work that votive objects could perform: terracotta figurines, for example, could function as a symbol of transformation (i.e. from wet, squishy clay to brittle orange ceramic), while wooden votives, with their physical traces of the chisel, could evoke connections not only to the artist's body, but also to the tree and even the landscape from which the wood had been taken.

What other things did votives touch, apart from the hands of their dedicants and makers? In the few instances where votives are found in situ of their original dedication, rather than in 'secondary' deposits such as purpose-dug pits within the sanctuary, we find them placed on altars, or around statue bases, as at the sites of Gravisca and Lavinium in Italy (Comella 1978; Fenelli 1975). Textual sources also indicate that ancient worshippers often strived to place their offering on or near to the cult statue. The Greek travel writer Pausanias describes statues that were completely obscured by the mass of votives attached to them, like the statue of Hygeia at the sanctuary of Titane which was covered by mountains of hair and 'Babylonian raiment' (variously translated as 'bandages' or 'ribbons'; Pausanias 2.11.6). At the sanctuary of Asklepios at Athens, miniature votive offerings were even placed in the hand of the cult statue; we know this from the evidence of inscribed inventories that were compiled in the second century BCE, which record 'eight sealstones and a *typos* [metal plaque]' in the hand of Asklepios (Aleshire 1991). Again, this desire to place offerings on or near to the miracle-working statue is not unique to Greco-Roman religion, and analogies can be found in many different faiths and geographical contexts. Some particularly compelling examples are discussed in Frank Graziano's recent study *Votive Offerings and Miraculous Images in Mexico*, where he describes worshippers touching the glass around sacred images and putting their tears into the glass coffins with the image of the dead Christ. He introduces the concept of 'proximity' as a counterpart to 'direct contact', commenting that the worshippers' desire to place votives as near to the holy image as possible (if not actually touching it) demonstrates that 'an image's power radiates, with diminishing concentration as one is distanced from the epicenter' (Graziano 2016: 77). Similar comments might be made of ancient cult statues – as we shall see further below.

DIVINE HEALING

The physical contact between a votive offering and cult statue can on some level be seen to represent the encounter between the bodies of the dedicant and deity (on the complexity of this relationship between votive and body see Graham, forthcoming). But some Greco-Roman worshippers did experience a more-or-less unmediated contact with the divine body. From the fifth century BCE onwards, sick people visited sanctuaries sacred to the healing god Asklepios, often sleeping there overnight in a ritual known as incubation (Renberg 2017). Written sources describe Asklepios as active in the sanctuary, wandering amongst his sleeping patients and curing them by using therapies that were largely tactile in nature. Some of our most detailed accounts come from the fourth century BCE *iamata* ('miracle') inscriptions from the Asklepios sanctuary at Epidauros in central Greece. These tales describe the god performing complex surgical operations such as the excision of diseased eyeballs, the sewing up of stomachs, and even the re-attaching of the severed head to the body (LiDonnici 1995). Other textual descriptions include the healing of the blind god Ploutos ('Wealth') in Aristophanes' comic play of that name. Here the god Asklepios sits down at Ploutos' head, takes out a purple rag and wipes the patient's eyelids – before summoning his two enormous snakes who disappear under the rag to lick Ploutos' eyes (*Ploutos* 410ff).

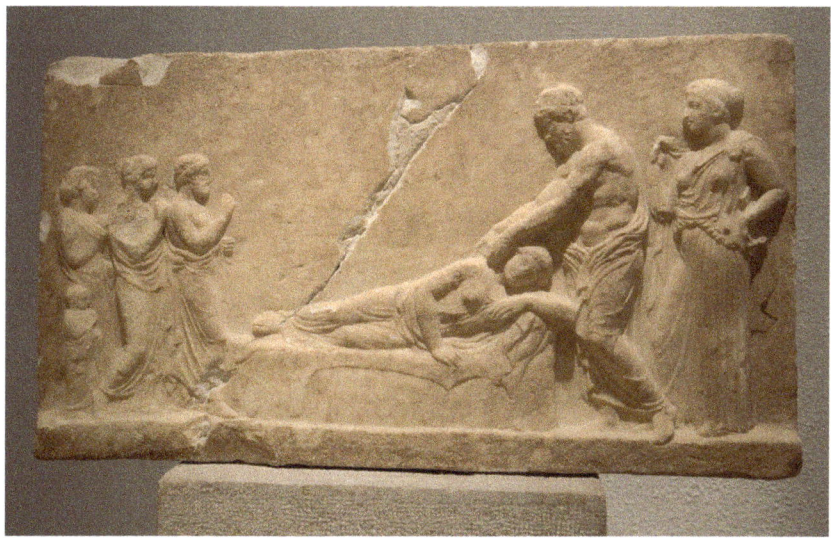

Figure 9.2 Marble votive relief showing Asklepios healing via touch, from the Asklepieion at Piraeus, c. 350 BCE. Piraeus Archaeological Museum (Art Resource ART370833).

Visual images also depict Asklepios in direct manual contact with a sleeping patient, like the marble relief in Figure 9.2, which comes from the sanctuary of Asklepios at Piraeus near Athens. This relief shows the muscular, bearded deity manipulating the body of his female patient, who reclines on a couch covered with the skin of an animal. The woman lies on her left side, her head resting in the crook of her arm while her elbow seems to dig into the god's knee. The god's outstretched arms form a continuous line with her reclining body, and present an image of balanced physical harmony. But the woman's awkwardly-posed form raises questions about the totality of her sensual experience. Is she asleep or awake? Can she feel (and smell) the animal fur beneath her, and the pressure of the unyielding stone couch against her arm and hips? What do the god's hands feel like as they press into her shoulder? Notably, this relief would have been displayed within the healing sanctuary, thereby providing an aspirational image for other worshippers who also hoped to feel the divine healing touch.

These images of sacred healing suggest two broader themes in ancient religious touching which resonate with the practices of sacred washing discussed earlier. One theme is *transformation*, since the contact with the divine healing hand or with the purificatory water sets in motion a fundamental (and apparently instantaneous) transformation within the human body. In healing, the sick body is transformed into a healthy one; in washing, the momentary contact with the water changes a polluted body into a pure one. The second theme concerns the 'visuality' of touch – that is, the way that the moment of tactile contact can be witnessed and scrutinised by external observers. As Susan Guettel Cole remarks: 'the gesture [of washing] was important because it would have signalled to other participants that anyone pure enough to touch the *perirrhanterion* was eligible to take part in a ceremony honouring the gods and would therefore not jeopardise either the ritual or the other participants.' The same applies to the Philadelphia law mentioned above, where the demonstrative touching of the inscribed stone provided a direct, unmistakable testimony of purity before the assembled masses. In this respect, the sense of touch differs from other senses like smell and hearing in which the sense-stimuli are invisible, and in which the moment of sensing remains entirely hermetic and inaccessible to outside viewers. To put this another way, while the female patient depicted in the relief at Figure 9.2 was experiencing an intensely personal and unique moment, it was nonetheless witnessed by the five other people depicted on the relief, as well as the 'external' viewers of the relief – who all thus knew exactly when the contact had happened, even if they would never know exactly *what it felt like*.

TOUCH IN ROMAN ASIA MINOR: THE 'CONFESSION' STELAI

While the objects and practices described so far could be found in many different regions of the Greco-Roman world, each classical sanctuary also had its own unique 'touchscape', in which these objects and practices were reconfigured to fit the local context. The second part of this chapter zooms in on some small rural sanctuaries in the Greek-speaking regions of Lydia and Phrygia, in the Roman-governed region of Asia Minor. Most of these sanctuaries have actually left little or no trace in the archaeological record, but hundreds of stone dedicatory inscriptions have been found in this area, many of which were reused as building materials in local Turkish villages. These inscriptions help us to reconstruct the basic appearance of the sanctuaries where they were originally displayed – as well as giving us some insight into the rich multisensory world inhabited by the people who dedicated them. My discussion will focus on a small group of around 150 inscriptions which were set up between the first and third century CE, and which are conventionally labelled 'confession inscriptions' or, more recently, 'reconciliation' or 'propitiatory' inscriptions (Petzl 1994; Chaniotis 1995, 2004, 2009; Gordon 2004; Rostad 2006). Written in a distinctly local Greek dialect, these inscriptions record a series of colourful ritual transgressions (*hamartia*), which had been committed by the dedicants or their family members, punished by the gods, and monumentalised in the form of a stele, to act as a warning to others.

Let us begin by looking at an example. Figure 9.3 is a drawing of a stele from southwest Mysia, which was dedicated in the first or second century CE by a man named Meidon. The stele is made from white-grey marble; its upper portion shows a pediment containing a rosette and decorated with palmette acroteria. A Greek inscription occupies the lower half of the stele, while the portion between the inscription and the pediment depicts an eagle standing on top of an altar. A disembodied human hand appears from the right of the scene and appears to offer something – perhaps a morsel of food – to the eagle (another possible interpretation is that it is *taking* the morsel from the eagle's beak: see Van Straten 1976).

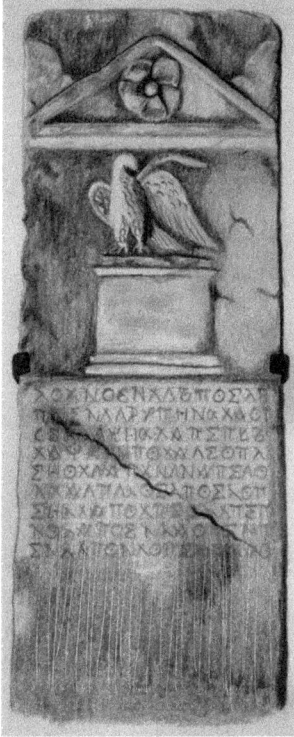

Figure 9.3 Stele of Meidon, from Mysia, first–second century CE. Marble, height 77 cm. Manisa Archaeological Museum, inv. no. 395. Drawing by Patricia Rodrigues de Souza.

The Greek inscription translates as follows:

> Meidon son of Menandros held a drinking party in the temple of Zeus Trosou, and his servants ate unsacrificed meat, and he [the god] made him dumb for three months and appeared to him in his dreams [so that he] set up a stela and inscribed on it what had befallen him, and [only] then did he begin to speak [again]. (Petzl 1994, no. 1; translation modified from Gordon 2004: 189)

Like most of the other confession stelai, this example begins with the narration of a transgression. In this case it was a double transgression, since Meidon had held a banquet in Zeus' temple *and* eaten meat that had not been sacrificed. The narrative then immediately moves on to record the punishment that was visited on the guilty Meidon, which involved him being 'struck dumb' for a period of three months. During this time the god appeared to Meidon in his dreams, leading him to set up the stele as an act of reparation, after which he was cured of his affliction. The chronology of these last events is slightly confusing in that the cure is only effected *after* the stele (describing the cure) is set up. It may actually be the case that two stelai were offered by Meidon, or that the inscription was wishful thinking. In any case, it seems likely that the figural image on this stele was interpreted as an allegorical representation of the propitiation, with the hand of Meidon making a food offering to the bird of Zeus.

The inscription provides the bare bones of this story. But in doing so, it opens up many more questions about Meidon's experience. When and how did this banquet take place? Was it after dark? Did Meidon and his friends sneak into the temple? Like many other of the dedicants of these stelai, Meidon himself may have been a *hierodoulos* ('sacred slave') who had a particularly close relationship with the god, and therefore perhaps greater access to the temple, as well as a heightened responsibility to respect that space. But why did Meidon hold the banquet here, and not elsewhere? Where did the meat come from? And was he the only one of his friends to be punished? Some extra details can tentatively be added from comparison with the other stelai. For instance, the epiphany of the god in a dream is quite common in the inscriptions, and may have been one of the ways that these worshippers were helped to identify the past transgression which had led to their suffering. Several scholars have suggested that the erection of the stele was accompanied by some kind of oral testimony spoken in the presence of an audience, which constituted a more ephemeral, performative supplement to the material gift of the stele (see e.g. Chaniotis 2009).

Most of the confession inscriptions follow the same pattern of transgression-punishment-reparation that we see in Meidon's stele, although many examples also include a statement of the god's power and greatness at the beginning or end of the narrative. The transgressions encompass a wide range of religious faults, including the failure to wash, to abstain from sex at the required times, to fulfil priestly duties, or to respect the property of the sanctuary. Meanwhile, the punishments consist of an array of physical ailments, referred to via the parts of the body (X was 'punished in his eyes', Y was 'punished on her buttocks'). There are also instances of mental illness and even death. Some inscriptions mention that a cure was granted before the stele was erected, but most do not, and it is likely that many stelai were set up in the hope of divine forgiveness and healing. In some cases, including those in which the transgressor had been punished with death (and so had no hope of receiving a cure), it seems that the stele was set up by the family members, who hoped to avoid any continued, inherited punishment that might arise from their connection with the guilty individual (see Hughes 2017a: ch. 5 for further discussion of this issue).

TRANSGRESSIVE TOUCH

The stele of Meidon hints at how these inscriptions might help us find out about ancient sensory experience and its relationship to religion. Meidon and his friends taste (and inevitably smell and touch) the pieces of meat; Meidon sees and hears the god in his dream; while the hand depicted in the relief touches the small offering, and perceives the distal touch of the eagle's beak as it pressed against that offering. Many of the other stelai contain equally rich detail about sensory engagements: so we read about people fighting, having sex, suffering pain, and we see them grasping onto wreaths, food sacrifices and sceptres (on which see further below). In scrutinising the stelai, I have identified three main tactile themes that run through the whole group of stories. However, this is not a comprehensive discussion, and touch – like all the other senses – would have featured in these experiences in multiple different ways, which were often unique to the dedicant's personal narrative.

The first theme is that of 'transgressive touch', which refers to the acts of touching which contravened ritual laws, and which were thus considered as forbidden and punishable. While none of the transgressions can be reduced to a single sensory component, there are some in which touch

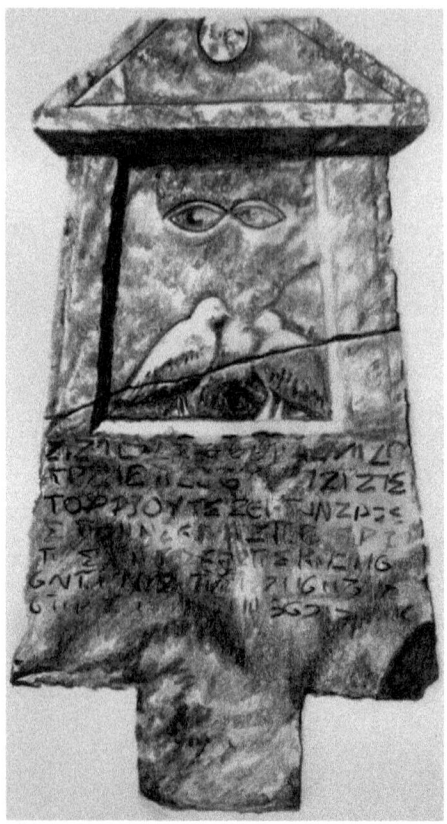

Figure 9.4 Stele of Diokles, showing the birds he stole and the eyes which were struck blind as punishment, from the sanctuary of Zeus Sabazios and Meter Hipta in Kula. White marble, height 66 cm. Drawing by Patricia Rodrigues de Souza.

plays a particularly central and definitive role. For instance, sexual intercourse occurs in several of the inscriptions, including one from the territory of Silandos in which a man named Theodorus admits to having sexual relations with three different women in the sanctuary before being punished by the gods 'on his eyes' (Petzl 1994: no. 5). Meanwhile, a number of stelai record acts of physical violence against the sanctuary or its property. A stele from Kollyda in Lydia reports how a mob carrying swords, sticks and stones entered a sanctuary during a festival, attacked the sacred slaves and broke divine images (Herrmann and Malay 2007: 110–113, no. 84; Chaniotis 2006: 143), while a dedicant from Mons Toma admits to cutting wood from the sacred grove of Zeus Didymeites (Petzl 1994: no. 10; cf. ibid.: no. 76 for another similar example).

Each of the stories described above revolves around a moment of tactual contact, which is often reflected in the main verbs of transgression ('holding', 'breaking', 'chopping'). And thinking seriously about the role played by touch in these stories can help us to imagine ourselves into the experience, as well as to identify new questions about the sequence and nature of events. The stele depicted at Figure 9.4 comes from the sanctuary of Zeus Sabazios and Meter Hipta in Kula, and it records the transgression of a man named Diokles. It reads: 'Because I caught the birds belonging to the divinities, I was punished in the eyes, and I inscribed on the stele the miraculous power of the gods.' The birds appear within a niche above the inscription, carved in high relief which contrasts with the engraved forms of the eyes above them (and the Greek letters below them). In fact, their bulging marble forms invite the viewer to reach out and touch – or at least to *imagine* touching them. Here, as in other cases, pondering the role of touch makes us think harder about what happened in this story, identifying gaps in the narrative as recounted in the written inscription. In this case, the ambiguity partly arises from the word 'caught' (*epeiasa*, probably a form of the verb *piezo*, which elsewhere in Greek sometimes is used to mean 'press tightly', to 'squeeze', even to 'distress'). Were the birds' feathery forms still moving when Diokles wrapped his fingers around them – or had he stunned or even killed the birds first? Did he carry them outside the sanctuary? And did he hold one in each hand, or are the two birds in the relief simply visual shorthand for a larger number of birds, captured (and perhaps 'squeezed') over a longer period of time?

Crucially, in the vast majority of cases, the tactile contact only becomes 'activated' as transgressive either because it occurs within the holy ground, or because it happens at the wrong (i.e. ritually forbidden) time. Wearing dirty garments, chopping trees, herding cattle, hunting birds – none of these acts would be considered wrong in other contexts. The confession inscriptions thus construct discrepant modes of touching within and beyond the border of the sanctuary, mobilising the sense of touch to ensure the spaces of ritual *felt different*, in some way, from quotidian life outside the sanctuary.

PUNITIVE TOUCH

The second major way in which the sense of touch pervades the confession stelai has to do with the divine punishments that were directed against the transgressive acts discussed above. As mentioned already, these punishments took the form of illness, which can be reframed here in terms of the suppression or accentuation of physical sensations – including, but not limited to, tactile sensations. The punitive *suppression* of the senses applies particularly to the several attested cases of blindness, including the story of Diokles that we have just met. In this stele (Figure 9.4), a pair of eyes is depicted above the pair of birds that Diokles stole – a clear visual device for representing causality between crime and punishment. Meanwhile, Meidon (Figure 9.3) was temporarily 'struck dumb', a punishment which may have involved the suppression of kinaesthetic movement (i.e. the quelling of the vocal chords) as well as of the sense of hearing (which is so closely related to speaking). A number of other inscriptions reveal that their dedicants had been placed by the gods into a 'death-like state' (*isothanatous*). This state would presumably have been experienced as a temporary suppression of *all* the senses – at least, that is probably how it appeared to outside observers. But did the punished person themselves actually cease to experience sensory stimuli? Or is this the ancient equivalent of a 'locked-in' syndrome, where the afflicted person appeared non-sensate to observers, but did in fact continue to hear, see and smell?

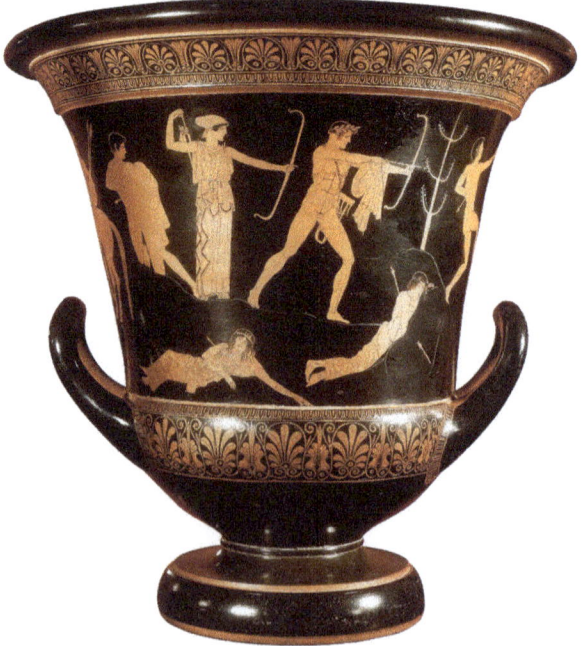

Figure 9.5 Calyx krater depicting Apollo and his sister Artemis killing the children of Niobe, from Orvieto, 460–450 BCE. Height 54 cm. Photograph: Getty Images.

While blindness, dumbness and 'death-like states' involved the suppression or dampening of perceptual sensations, other types of punishments involved *heightened* sensory experiences in the form of illnesses and pain. The bodily afflictions mentioned or depicted in the stele included illnesses of the buttocks, legs, genitals, arms and breasts, which have invited the retrospective diagnosis of conditions like tumours, gout and mastitis. Today, neuroscientists and philosophers tend to consider pain as distinctive from touch, partly on account of its 'intransitive' nature, and the existence in the body of a discrete nocioceptive system. As Matthew Fulkerson writes, '[Pain scenarios] are not paradigm instances of tactual perception, and if they seem more closely tied to touch, then this is something in need of explanation' (Fulkerson 2016). In classical antiquity, however, illness and pain *were* commonly envisaged as resulting from the touch of the gods – or, rather, from the touch of the gods' weapons or sidekicks, since the gods were not described or depicted as wounding mortal bodies with their own bare hands. Greek mythology gives us the examples of Apollo and Artemis raining down arrows on the children of Niobe (Figure 9.5), Zeus

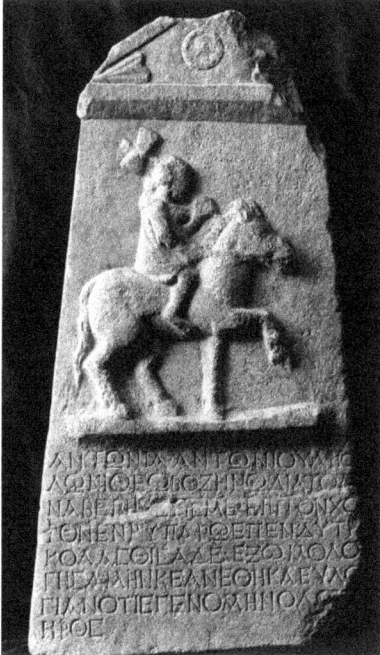

Figure 9.6 Stele depicting Apollo Bozenos with his axe, from Kula. Height 71 cm. Staatl Museum Berlin (Inv. no. Sk 680). Photograph reproduced courtesy of bpk images.

shooting his thunderbolt, Artemis sending her hounds to ravage the body of Actaeon, and Dionysus instructing his maenads to rip Pentheus apart. Such paradigmatic images of divinely-inflicted pain would have given sick people an imaginative template into which they could place their own suffering – whether or not this meant that they *literally* attributed their aches, itches and burns to the unseen arrows of the gods.

The stele depicted in Figure 9.6 is particularly relevant here, since it shows Apollo Bozenos holding his characteristic attribute of the double-axe, as he rides across the relief on his horse. This stele was dedicated by a woman named Antonia whose crime was wearing a dirty gown: she writes that '(I), Antonia, daughter of Antonius, (dedicate) this stela to the god Apollo of Boza because I went up to the dance [or perhaps the "place" = ?temple] in a dirty robe, and, being punished, have made my confession...' (Petzl 1994: no. 43; translation by Richard Gordon, who also makes the connection between the axe and divine punishment: Gordon 2004: 185). As in many of the other inscriptions the punishment is indicated verbally by a form of the verb *kolazein*, which means 'to punish' (note that the other commonly-used word for punishment in the inscriptions is *nemezein*, the root of our 'nemesis'). These non-specific terms leave the mode of punishment open to the imagination, although in Antonia's stele the image of the axe provides a powerful visual cue. In another stele, a sickle appears as an instrument of divine punishment; this is the long inscription from Kula recounting the story of a woman named Tatias, whose crime was that of making a false judicial prayer (Petzl 1994: no. 69, dated 156 CE). We hear how

> for this reason, the gods exercised a punishment which she did not escape. Similarly, her son Sokrates, when he was passing by the entrance which leads to the grove, having a sickle in his hands with which one cuts down vines, the sickle fell on his foot, and thus he died within a day, suffering his punishment. The gods at Aziotta are great!

We should note that this accident happened when Sokrates was just outside the entrance to the sacred grove, thus recalling Frank Graziano's words about power and proximity cited earlier in this chapter. Was it the case that the god's power was particularly intense in this spot in the landscape? Or was the location simply intended to underline the fact that this accident had a divine origin? Whatever the answer, Sokrates' perception that a god was somehow behind his suffering cannot fail to have shaped his experience of the wound, and his gradual death over the next few hours.

TOUCHING THINGS: WHERE MORTAL AND DIVINE HANDS MEET

The third touch-related theme raised by the stelai concerns material objects that are touched by both divine and mortal hands. As a prelude, it is useful to remember that in Greco-Roman art and literature, gods and goddesses are very often depicted as holding things – whether this be weapons (see Figures 9.1, 9.5 and 9.6), tridents, eagles, bags, crowns, thunderbolts, sceptres, lyres, cups, flowers or statuettes. This propensity of the classical gods for holding things must partly be due to the requirements of an anthropomorphic representational system which needed to distinguish between mortals and gods, as well as to accommodate multiple deities. It is true that there are other visual devices which also help to distinguish between divine (and mortal) bodies: for instance relative size, as well as colour and 'dazzle' or 'shine'. Nevertheless, the easiest way of distinguishing mortals and gods – and of correctly identifying a god as, say, Zeus rather than Poseidon – was via the things they touched – their

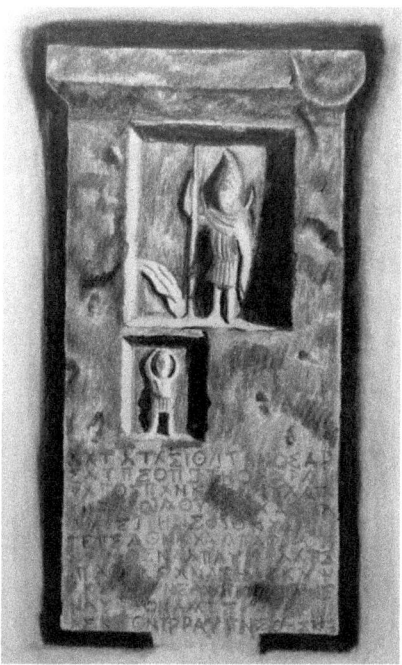

Figure 9.7 Confession stele showing the god Men holding a sceptre, from the territory of Saittai in Lydia, 164–165 CE. Drawing by Patricia Rodrigues de Souza.

attributes – which were so fundamental to their identity that they could even replace the deity's body itself (cf. the eagle in Figure 9.3).

Returning to the confession stelai, we find various objects in the hands of the gods, including pine cones, crowns and sceptres. This last object is a tall stick that is shown standing upright on the ground, forming a parallel line with the god's body. The sceptre appears in at least half a dozen stelai, including nos. 3, 52, 58, 61, 67 and 68 of Georg Petzl's 1994 catalogue. Figure 9.7 shows one example, in which the god Men, who wears the Phrygian hat and cloak, holds the sceptre in one hand and cradles a small object (identified by some commentators as a pine-cone) in the other. Reading through the inscriptions on these stelai, it becomes clear that sceptres had a very specific meaning in these areas of Asia Minor. Several inscriptions refer to the 'raising' of a *skeptron* by local residents and priests; in each case, this action appears to be one element of a formal judicial prayer, issued in response to a crime committed by another mortal. The precise mechanics of the *skeptron* ritual are unclear, but it seems likely that an injured person went to the temple, and – with the help of priests who are often represented in the reliefs – recited prayers, and raised the *skeptron*, which may have been placed on a base near to or even inside the temple. As Henk Versnel notes (1991: 76), this was 'a question of making visible the present power of the god', who was summoned to intervene in human affairs. At this point, the divinity was entrusted with identifying the culprit (if their identity was not yet known) and punishing them. Once this happened, the culprit would need to make reparation, which might take the form of giving back the stolen property and/or paying a fine. After the wrongdoer had been punished, had confessed and set up a stele, the sceptre could be taken down (*luthenai to skeptron*) and the judicial prayer thereby 'dissolved'.

These judicial procedures have been the topic of long debates. But in the present context, the most significant factor is one that has not yet been discussed: that is, the materiality of the *skeptron*, and its use as a device to link mortals and gods via asynchronous touch. Although we do not know much about the appearance and feel of this object (although we might guess that it was carved from wood), the materiality of the sceptre – its physical continuity through time and space – would have enabled it to function as a site of encounter between the hands of gods and the hands of mortal women and men. This encounter was ultimately indirect and asynchronous: first, the sceptre was touched (whether caressed, squeezed or rubbed) by the devotee at the time of the dedication; then, presumably after the dedicant had left the sanctuary, the sceptre was picked up by the god, who contemplated it and tested its weight (and the metaphorical weight of the accusation) before planting it once more into the holy ground.

This idea of the 'twice-touched' sceptre opens up a new dimension for how we imagine religious material culture to work. While we tend to discuss objects in ancient sanctuaries in visual terms (offerings, for instance, are routinely described as being intended for gods to 'look at' and 'read', as well as being 'visual testimony' of the god's healing power) sight was certainly not the only sense that could be used to apprehend and understand these sacred items. As we have just seen, classical culture was full of images of touching, feeling gods, who appeared grasping objects and attributes on pots and reliefs, or took on three-dimensional form in the cult statues that were then piled with offerings. And I would argue that, collectively, these images of *gods touching things* offered devotees a blueprint of divine behaviour which could easily be transferred to their own votive gifts and dedications. In other words, a woman who brought a garment to the sanctuary could then easily imagine the goddess caressing the fabric, contemplating the shape and size of its erstwhile wearer, before folding it again neatly to put back amongst the other offerings she had received that day. And the man who rubbed his thumb across the face of a silver figurine could imagine the deity taking it into his hands too – testing its weight in his palm, even biting gently into the shining body to test the purity of the precious metal, and to taste the salty residue from the dedicant's mortal palm.

For the givers of votives, then, this expectation of divine handling led to a sense of added closeness with the deity, and a degree of intimacy that would have been lacking from a distant, purely visual contemplation of the votive gift. This is partly to do with the individualisation of experience: a god who (only) gazes upon his offerings does not necessarily focus on each one in turn, but a god who picks up an offering and rotates it in his hands *does* single that gift out, even if just for a moment. This physical intimacy has important overlaps with knowledge, which again is a theme that Amy Whitehead will pick up and explore further in the next chapter of this volume. Suffice it to say here that writers, artists and scientists have all emphasised in different ways how far tactile experience of objects can lead to a qualitatively different understanding, often (but not always) working together with vision and the other senses to allow deep 'cross-modal' appreciations. For the ancient dedicant, one of the votive's most powerful functions may have been to make themself better known to the god – a god who interacted with all the unique multisensory qualities of the offering, including the tactile properties of weight, temperature and texture.

CONCLUSION

This chapter has explored some of the ways in which the sense of touch operated in ancient Greco-Roman sanctuaries. It began by looking at some of the most common types of classical sacred touch, identifying certain overarching themes like transformation, healing, and the close relationship between touch and vision (thus echoing the discussion of Byzantine icons by Angeliki Lymberopoulou in Chapter 5 of this volume). After this, I zoomed in on an area of the Roman Empire where touch seems to have been at a particularly high premium – the scattered rural sanctuaries of Greek-speaking Asia Minor. Here I used the so-called confession inscriptions to identify three important ways in which the sense of touch permeated religious life: first, by policing forbidden actions; second, by the administering of divine punishment; and third, by the use of mediating objects to enable the asynchronous touching of divine and mortal bodies.

Finally, I argued that this last point about mediating objects has a broader significance for the study of ancient material religion, since it forces us to recognise the extent to which the Greco-Roman gods were not simply 'watchful', but also 'grasping'. Here my argument drew both on the evidence of objects left in sanctuaries, *and* on the rich world of classical myth, particularly as it is communicated through the visual arts. In the modern world, myth and ritual have traditionally been studied in relative isolation; however, the theme of touch (and in fact sensory experience in general) indicates one way in which these two major spheres of ancient life might be woven together again. In this case, I suggested that the countless mythical images of 'gods holding things' provided an imaginative template which could shape the ancient devotee's own expectations of religious experience. Myth informed worshippers that the deities were highly tactile beings, who moved around, picked things up and held them in their hands for long periods. Surely this could not fail to have consequences for the ways in which people thought about the objects they used in ritual – the things they left behind them, as darkness fell on the sanctuary?

REFERENCES

Aleshire, S. B. 1991. *Asklepios at Athens: Epigraphic and Prosopographic Essays on the Athenian Healing Cults*. Amsterdam: Gieben.

Chaniotis, A. 1995. 'Illness and Cures in the Greek Propitiatory Inscriptions and Dedications of Lydia and Phrygia' in H. F. J. Horstmanshoff, P. J. van der Eijk and

P. H. Schrijvers (eds), *Ancient Medicine in its Socio-Cultural Context II*. Amsterdam: Rodopi. pp. 323–344.

Chaniotis, A. 2004. 'Under the Watchful Eyes of the Gods: Aspects of Divine Justice in Hellenistic and Roman Asia Minor' in S. Colvin (ed.), *The Greco-Roman East: Politics, Culture, Society*. Cambridge: Cambridge University Press. pp. 1–43.

Chaniotis, A. 2006. 'Rituals between Norms and Emotions: Rituals as Shared Experience and Memory' in E. Stavrianopoulou (ed.), *Ritual and Communication in the Graeco-Roman World*. Liège: Presses univeritaires de Liege. pp. 211–238. https://doi.org/10.4000/books.pulg.1144

Chaniotis, A. 2009. 'Ritual Performances of Divine Justice: The Epigraphy of Confession, Atonement, and Exaltation in Roman Asia Minor' in H. M. Cotton, R. G. Hoyland, J. J. Price and D. J. Wasserstein (eds), *From Hellenism to Islam: Cultural and Linguistic Change in the Roman Near East*. Cambridge: Cambridge University Press. pp. 115–153. https://doi.org/10.1017/CBO9780511641992.007

Cole, S. G. 2004. *Landscapes, Gender, and Ritual Space: The Ancient Greek Experience*. Berkeley: University of California Press. https://doi.org/10.1525/california/9780520235441.001.0001

Comella, A. 1978. *Il materiale votivo tardo di Gravisca*. Rome: Bretschnieder.

Dent, P. (ed.) 2014. *Sculpture and Touch*. London and New York: Routledge.

Draycott, J., and Graham, E.-J. 2017. *Bodies of Evidence: Ancient Anatomical Votives Past, Present and Future*. New York: Routledge.

Fenelli, M. 1975. 'Votivi anatomici' in *Lavinium II, Le tredici Are*. Rome: De Luca. pp. 206–252.

Fulkerson, M. 2016. 'Touch', *The Stanford Encyclopedia of Philosophy*. Online at https://plato.stanford.edu/archives/spr2016/entries/touch/ (accessed July 2017).

Ginouvès, R. 1962. *Balaneutikè. Recherches sur le bain dans l'antiquité grecque*. Paris: De Boccard.

Gordon, R. L. 2004. 'Raising a Sceptre: Confession Narratives from Lydia and Phrygia', *Journal of Roman Archaeology* 17: 177–196. https://doi.org/10.1017/S1047759400008217

Graham, E.-J. (forthcoming). 'Hand in "Hand"? Rethinking Anatomical Votives as Material Things' in V. Gasparini, M. Patzelt, R. Raja, A-K. Rieger, J. Rüpke and E. Urciuoli (eds), *Lived Religion in the Ancient Mediterranean World: Approaching Religious Transformations from Archaeology, History and Classics*. Berlin: De Gruyter.

Graziano, F. 2016. *Votive Offerings and Miraculous Images in Mexico*. Oxford: Oxford University Press. https://doi.org/10.1093/acprof:oso/9780199790869.001.0001

Hermann, P., and Malay, H. 2007. *New Documents from Lydia, Tituli Asiae Minoris*. Vienna: Ergänzungsband.

Hughes, J. 2017a. *Votive Body Parts in Greek and Roman Religion*. Cambridge: Cambridge University Press. https://doi.org/10.1017/9781316662403

Hughes, J. 2017b. 'Souvenirs of the Self: Personal Belongings as Votive Offerings in Ancient Religion', *Religion in the Roman Empire* 3.2: 181–201.

LiDonnici, L. R. 1995. *The Epidaurian Miracle Inscriptions: Text, Translation, and Commentary*. Atlanta: Scholars Press.

Paoletti, O. 2005. 'Mondo Greco' in *ThesCRA* Vol. II. Los Angeles: Getty Publications. pp. 3–33.

Parker, R. 1983. *Miasma: Pollution and Purification in Early Greek Religion*. Oxford: Clarendon Press.
Petzl, G. 1994. *Die Beichtinschriften Westkleinasiens*. Bonn: Rudolf Habelt.
Renberg, G. H. 2017. *Where Dreams May Come: Incubation Sanctuaries in the Greco-Roman World*. Leiden: Brill.
Rostad, A. 2006. *Human Transgression – Divine Retribution: A Study of Religious Transgressions and Punishments in Greek Cultic Regulations and Lydian-Phrygian Reconciliation Inscriptions*, PhD thesis, University of Bergen, available online at http://bora.uib.no/handle/1956/2026.
Shaya, J. 2005. 'The Greek Temple as Museum: The Case of the Legendary Treasure of Athena from Lindos', *American Journal of Archaeology* 109.3: 423–442. https://doi.org/10.3764/aja.109.3.423
Sokolowski, F. 1955. *Lois sacrées de l'Asie Mineure*. Paris: de Boccard.
Van Straten, F. T. 1976. 'Daikrates' Dream. A Votive Relief from Kos and Some Other Kat'onar Dedications', *BABesch* 51: 1–38.
Versnel, H. 1991. 'Beyond Cursing: The Appeal to Justice in Judicial Prayers' in C. A. Faraone and D. Obbink (eds), *Magika Hiera: Ancient Greek Magic and Religion*. Oxford: Oxford University Press. pp. 60–106.

Jessica Hughes is a Senior Lecturer in Classical Studies at The Open University, UK. She works on material religion, classical reception studies and the cultural history of the Italian region of Campania. She has recently published the monograph *Votive Body Parts in Greek and Roman Religion* (Cambridge University Press, 2017) and is currently researching material religion and cultural memory at the Catholic Shrine of the Blessed Virgin of the Rosary in Pompeii.

Chapter 10

Touching, Crafting, Knowing:
Religious Artefacts and the Fetish within Animism

AMY WHITEHEAD

It was a hot July day in 2007 when I first entered the Sanctuary of the Virgin of Alcala de los Gazules in the province of Cadiz in Andalusia, Spain. Typically Andalusian in architectural style, the shrine complex was whitewashed, and a mini-paradise of plants and birds inhabited the tiled patio area within the walls of the *Hermita*. Two dark, heavy, mediaeval-looking doors gave access to the shrine off to one side of the patio which required visitors to step up, and in. Stepping over the threshold and coming out of the sun, it took a few seconds for the shrine and its contents to come into focus. It was, however, in these few seconds before I could see clearly that my senses began to collectively engage my surroundings. I could smell a mixture of flowers and frankincense. I could feel the coolness of stone and marble, and I noticed failed attempts at silence (the sounds of footsteps and parents hushing small children were audible). And once my eyes finally adjusted, I saw the focus of all this activity. Elevated above the main altar, in a chamber of her own and wearing what appeared to be a heavy gold-embroidered mantle, I saw the small wooden statue of the Virgin of Alcala (Figure 10.1). Only about three feet tall, she was standing, crowned in gold, on a thick marble pedestal (as I imagine she still stands now) holding court within the walls of her sanctuary as she has done for at least the last 600 years (or more). Further, I noticed that there were people behind the Virgin, and to my surprise I saw that the statue was 'accessible' via a set of winding stairs that goes from the ground up to her chamber. This, I told myself, would certainly not have been the case in the more northerly European climes from which I come. Religious statues in the UK are also placed on pedestals, but they are usually cordoned off. The smallness of this Virgin with her delicate European features did not appear to reflect the magnitude of her presence, nor, as I was soon to learn, the complexity involved in the goings-on of this vernacular Catholic religiosity.

I had begun my doctoral research in 'material religion' the previous year. Inspired by this timely encounter with the Virgin of Alcala, and with permission given by the village priest and *Santero* (the shrine caretaker), I embarked on a four-year programme of investigative, qualitative, participant observation research at and around the shrine. Accounts soon revealed that the statue of this Spanish Virgin is particularly powerful. Evidenced in the presence of baby paraphernalia placed strategically throughout the shrine, she is known in particular for her ability to cure infertility. According to devotees she 'feeds the hungry' through shrine-generated revenue and this includes the taking in and of feeding stray animals (several cats and dogs live at the shrine and are often seen around the doors). She is also known to heal the sick and to save the lives of those who have been in road traffic and other accidents that take place in close proximity to the shrine. Dried bloodied hospital bandages, locks of hair given as 'promises', and gold rings (usually family heirlooms) on the fingers of the statue can be seen. Significant, too, are the hundreds of painted *ex-votos* that line the walls of this working shrine, all of which provide a living, volatile record that attests to the many miracles stated above, as well as to Virgin's power, and the love, healing and protection she demonstrates toward her devotees and the people of Alcala. As Jessica Hughes' chapter in this book reflects, this type of statue devotion and usages of votives can also be found in the ancient Greco-Roman world.

In both day-to-day activities and more ritualised religious performances, the Virgin receives physical affection from her devotees that is not entirely different from the ways in which some humans treat other humans who hold positions of noble, royal or higher social standing. For example, she is bathed, dressed, sung to and cared for by her own group of elite female caretakers called *camaristas* who form a significant part of her cult. Although parishioners chose to have their weddings, funerals and baptisms at the shrine, it is not a church. The churches are in the village of Alcala, some seven kilometres from the shrine. The priest, however, oversees the management of the shrine and selects the mantles that the Virgin will wear at different points in the liturgical calendar. The Virgin is displayed in such a way that devotees have regular access to her, and to her mantle, the 'thing' that provides the medium through which most physical interactions and negotiations take place. These interactions whereby

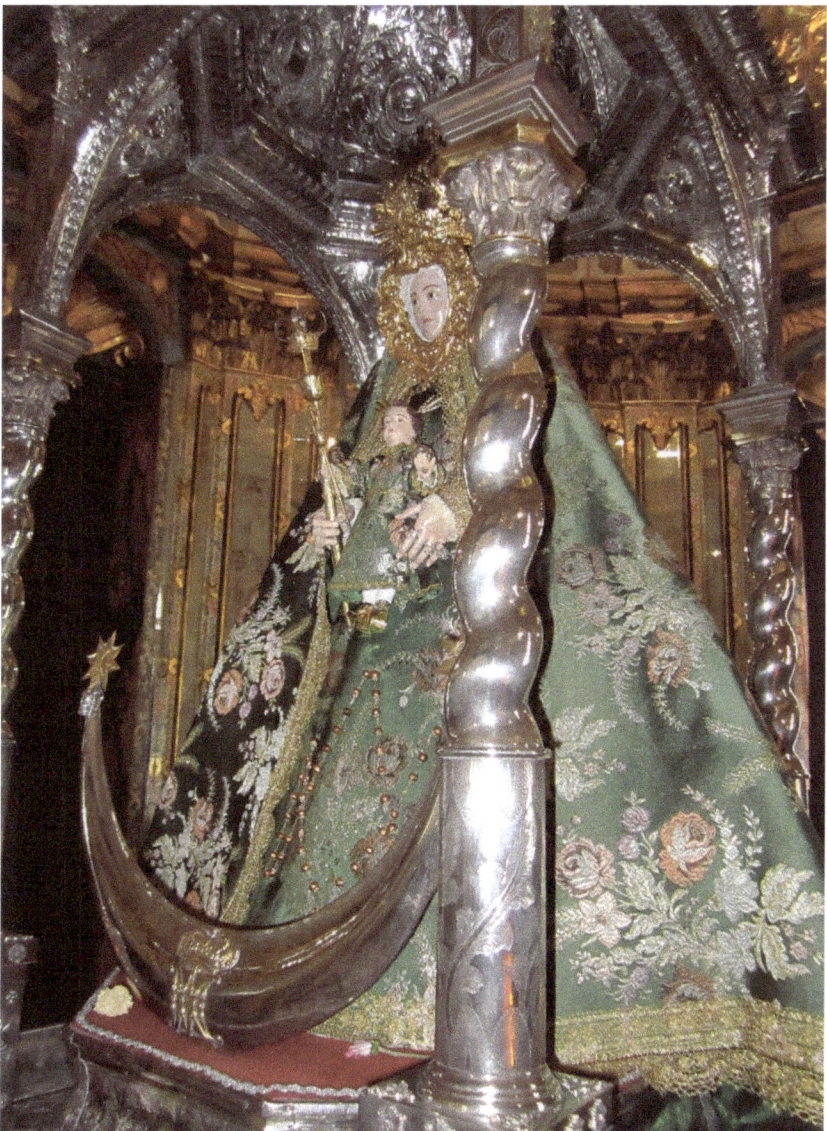

Figure 10.1 The Virgin of Alcala. Photograph by Amy Whitehead.

a devotee places the train of the Virgin's mantle over his/her head are some of the most intimate encounters that devotees can have with her. Here, cloaked in the semi-darkness provided by the heaviness of the mantle, notes and other small gifts can be gleaned whereby expressions of adoration, doubt, worry, thanks and faith are visibly manifest. Touching the Virgin, being touched by the Virgin, creating and giving gifts that are in different ways in touch with the Virgin, actively facilitate and co-creatively reinforce the relationships that exist between devotees and the statue.

Based on a combination of fieldwork observations and theoretical premises drawn from this small-scale study at Alcala, this chapter asserts that 'touch' is not only an intrinsic part of religion, but the principal facilitating medium through which religion, religious encounters and performances take place. The dynamics of 'touch' in relation to the statue of the Virgin will be explored using two interrelated themes: 'animism' and 'the fetish'. Using practical evidences, these relational discourses highlight the ways in which powerful religious artefacts are forged from raw materials, the significance of creativity, display and ritual performances, and how 'persons' (human and other-than-human) emerge ontologically from encounters. This first theme builds on a discussion of relationality applied to matter (Whitehead 2013a) and the 'new animism' (Harvey 2005a), and asserts that religious statues and devotees bring each other into co-creative, co-relational forms of being in moments of active relational engagement. This is exemplified through discussions about the gendered ritual performances involved in the caretaking practices surrounding the Virgin's powerful statue-body, alongside the dynamics involved in 'crafting', 'creativity' and the 'materials of the materiality' (Ingold 2011). These ideas serve as foundation to the second theme which, building on Graeber's 'fetish zone' (2005: 432), explores the productive, critical uses of the fetish within animism and evokes a 'relational zone'. Particularly useful when addressing the discourses surrounding religious material and performance cultures, the fetish is understood here as both 'object' and 'action'. It is used to explore the roles of the Virgin's mantle and the offerings she receives, asserting that both offerings and the mantle are extensions of both the statue and devotees. Further inspired by Johnson's (2000) critical use of the fetish in verb-form, e.g. 'to fetish', the chapter places the performances of 'touch' and 'fetish' on a relational continuum. These examinations demonstrate yet another dimension to 'touch' that further adds to discussions about the nature of religion, religious artefacts, creativity and the power inherent in matter. 'To fetish' is both to apprehend with the senses and to be invited into creative religious, relational action. 'To touch' is 'to fetish'.

MATERIAL RELIGION, PERFORMANCE AND TOUCH

Scholars such as King (2005) and Smith (2005) have rightly argued that what we call 'religion' should be approached on its own terms and not as a *sui generis* category. It can, however, be asserted that the one thing that all religions do have in common is an observable 'fact': all religionists 'do' religion in some form or other, and that 'doing' involves 'touch'. Just as all humans are 'material' and connected to this earthly realm, so are religions. How can it be conceived of otherwise? The only thing that separates religionists from the things that they 'do' is the *idea* that what they are doing is symbolic or representational and therefore points to something greater. Yet the problem lies in the fact that the significances of the things that religionists 'touch' and 'do' are often lost to the privileging of transcendence over immanence, subjects over objects, representations over 'the real thing', and spirit over matter, under which lies the assertion that 'true' religion can only occupy the abstract spaces of metaphysics and 'belief'. Further, within these mostly Protestant and academic discourses, religious objects (statues, offerings) and their materials (wood, bone, hair and stone) are often perceived as 'other', e.g. foreign and unknown, things that are treated with suspicion that must be controlled, mastered, undermined and relegated to the status of metaphor. A direct legacy of Greek thought and Plato's 'ideal forms', this 'problem of materiality' is also responsible for the privileging of official versions of what religion 'should be' over what it actually is: earthy, real, practical and functional. This chapter, however, approaches religion from the ground up. As it is understood here, religion is a volatile occurrence that literally *takes place* geographically in specific locales and consists of a variety of activities, ideas, traditions, materialities and performances that inevitably involve 'touch' along with the other four senses. Religion is understood here as 'material'.

In predominantly Catholic countries such as Spain, especially in the region of Andalusia, the most vibrant and passionate performances that take place in relation to Marian statues (the Virgin of Alcala being only one of many) are exercised most regularly through acts of 'touch' (Boissevain 1992). These acts include the giving of gifts/offerings, going beneath (and kissing) the Virgin's mantle (Figure 10.2; or if a family member has a baby, the baby is passed under the mantle in order to *conocer*, or 'know/meet', the Virgin), preparing and giving food from the money generated within the shrine and on the Virgin's behalf, and processing the statue in celebration of 'her day' (often referred to as her birthday). 'Touch', of course, can be understood in different ways. We can refer to the sense of touch or to the action of touch, or both. Our skin (the largest organ of the human body) is continually in a position of touch with its environment and surroundings, and, while sending messages to our brains, our sense of touch continually gathers millions of bits of information that help us apprehend and make sense of our worlds. Touch also helps humans establish social bonds. According to Serres, 'Pure touch gives access to information, a soft correlate of what was once called the intellect' (2008: 83). To touch something is to gain knowledge of it, or to know it, and the knowledge gained through 'touch' can be referred to as 'full-bodied' knowledge. This is certainly true of 'religious' or devotional knowledge/knowing. Touch-informed knowledge, as Serres suggests, is not oriented toward the mind exclusively; it requires the participation of the sum of all our parts. In terms of religious contexts where statues sit at the hearts of communities such as that of Alcala, both the sense of touch and the action of touching the statue are vital to religious tradition and continuation.

The Virgin is touched regularly and in a rich variety of both 'everyday' and more highly ritualised traditions and performances. A final but

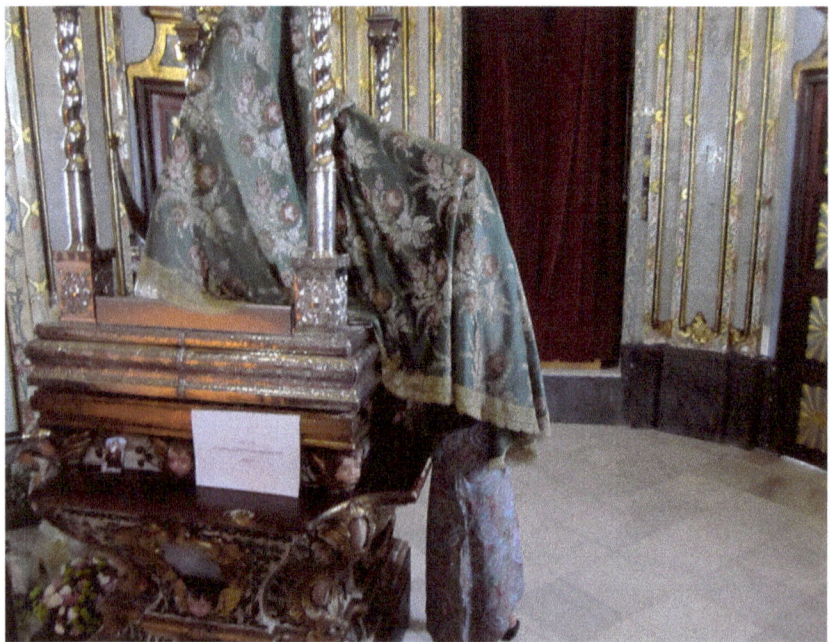

Figure 10.2 'Going under the mantle' of the Virgin of Alcala. Photograph by Jose Maria Estudillo de la Corte.

significant point in this section is that when devotees speak with, touch and give offerings to their Virgin, the acts are not symbolic but 'real'. The actions involved in the Virgin's care, for example, are not 'pretend' or, as Gell says, 'make believe' (1998: 134). Addressing the 'problem of idolatry', Gell tells us that

> The essence of idolatry is that it permits real physical interactions to take place between persons and divinities. To treat such interactions as 'symbolic' is to miss the point. (1998: 135)

Gell is right. Many academics have the tendency to place both religious object-oriented performances such as 'touch', as well as so-called objects such as statues themselves, into the abstract and safe categories of symbolism and representation. 'Agency' is another term that has somewhat contradictorily been used by Gell and others to describe that which occurs when devotees are in the presence of religious statues – such as episodes of *darśan*. This is exemplified in the commonly held position that humans 'give' or 'attribute' agency to objects. Yet, according to Leach (2007: 183), Gell's notion of agency is but another form of representation. These 'human-centred' positions also miss the point. Devotional encounters are, as this chapter suggests, not dualistic but 'full-bodied' sensual affairs that are performed most commonly through the fusing acts of touch. To categorically break down the parts of the whole (mind, matter, meaning) provides a weakened view that misrepresents the passion with which encounters often take place. In support of this, Barad suggests that 'matter and meaning are not separate elements. They are inextricably fused together, and no event, no matter how energetic, can tear them asunder' (2007: 3). This view relies on quantum physics to reveal the 'real nature' of matter. Applied to 'religious matter' such as the Virgin, it can be argued that modernist dualistic categories that separate subject from object are indeed impoverished.

The emotional quality or the sincerity of all devotees/practitioners is not, however, measurable, nor is the degree to which devotional encounters are ritually 'authentic' (Gade 2015: 81). Researchers must also be aware of the pitfalls of conducting qualitative research whereby devotees and others might embellish claims. Yet even these uncertainties are demonstrative of the volatile, relational terrain upon which we are treading. Practical evidences found in twenty-first century religions such as that of the cult of the Virgin of Alcala mean that rituals where statues are touched and/or treated as persons can no longer be considered merely symbolic gestures that signify something other than what they are: powerful, 'embodied' expressions of devotion that are capable of facilitating, maintaining and renewing relationships within religious contexts. Lived religion is, as this chapter will demonstrate, generative, messy and necessarily engaged in a variety of performances that operate within varying levels of emotional sincerity that involve touching and being in touch with forms of religious material expression, the dynamics of which will be here explored in relation to the overarching critical discourses of animism and the fetish.

ANIMISM: PERSONHOOD, CRAFTING AND CARETAKING

Personhood

De Witte tells us that '...touch is a powerful medium of religious communication, not only between human beings, but also between humans and spirits' (2015: 262). The performance of touch, however, not only mediates between 'humans and spirits', but also between human persons and 'other-than-human persons' such as religious statues. It serves as a momentary fusing agent that blurs existing ontological boundaries between subjects and objects, persons and things, making them questionable at least and contestable at best. Examples that present accounts of caretaking and crafting support this chapter's assertion that the ways in which the Virgin of Alcala is 'touched' is a prime indictor of her 'personhood'. This idea builds on Harvey's (2005a) newer usage of animism (as opposed to Tylor's [1871] animism) which suggests that the world is full of persons, only some of whom are human. That usage is not so much concerned with how persons come into being as it is with how those persons are to be behaved toward:

> The newer usage [of animism] refers to a concern with knowing how to behave appropriately towards persons, not all of whom are human. It refers to the widespread indigenous and increasingly popular 'alternative' understanding that humans share this world with a wide range of persons, only some of whom are human (Harvey 2005b: xi).

The notion of 'other-than-human persons' comes from Hallowell's (1960) interpretation of the Ojibwe understanding that 'persons' exist all around us. This idea is not anthropocentric, but inclusive of the objects, artefacts and the other beings who comprise the 'living world'. Thus building on Harvey (2005a) and Hallowell (1960), the term/concept of 'personhood' is being engaged here not only to address the treatment of religious objects such as the Virgin of Alcala, but also the ways in which she, and her devotees, come into co-inspired relational forms of ontological being during moments of active engagement which involve physical contact. In other words, the Virgin of Alcala may not be a 'person' all of the time; but her personhood (like that of other objects found in the shrine), emerges upon her being 'touched'.

'Touch', of course, goes both ways. Since 'touch' has the power to generate relationships, it can be argued that the practice of touch provides tangible evidences that 'persons' (statue-persons and human-persons) are coming into being and intersubjectivity is taking place. If I am touching either the statue of the Virgin or her mantle (discussed further along as an extension of her), then she/it is also touching me. This can be considered through what Serres refers to as 'co-mingling bodies':

> The skin is a variety of contingency: in it, through it, with it, the world and my body touch each other, the feeling and the felt, it defines their common edge. Contingency means common tangency: in it the world and the body intersect and caress each other. I do not wish to call the place in which I live a medium, I prefer to say that things mingle with each other and that I am no exception to that, I mix with the world which mixes with me. Skin intervenes between several things in the world and makes them mingle. (2008: 80)

As 'moderns' who are accustomed to understanding the world through the divisions that comprise the previously discussed constructs of subjects and objects, nature and culture, mind over matter, the idea that our bodies constantly co-mingle with our surroundings might come as a surprise. This angle places the physical interactions between the Virgin and her devotees on a relational continuum and supports the assertion that 'persons' come into forms of co-inspired being when human skin touches wooden skin, and wooden skin touches human skin. Here, once-estranged 'others' are made familiar and known through touch, and statue-bodies and human-bodies co-mingle and are momentarily inseparable.

Crafting

'Crafting' is explored here as another dimension of 'touch' that opens up a unique set of investigative issues and engages questions not only about the material properties of objects and the creativity involved in their making, but the social relations that are crafted when religious devotees interact with 'artefacts'. As I have argued elsewhere (Whitehead 2013a, 2013b), power relations exist in the context of the Virgin of Alcala whereby devotees and the statue maintain each other's positions through a kind of respectful tension; devotees 'need' the statue to be the central focus of village life as she has been for several hundred years. They need her protection, her 'mothering', her miracles and her power. She is also significant for providing the village with its local identity, and for helping the village to generate revenue. Equally, it can be suggested that the statue (who is vulnerable to deterioration if not conserved) relies on her devotees to keep her statue-body in a good condition, to bathe her, to sing to her, to take her on processions and to give her gifts. Graeber contributes to theories of social creativity by reimagining the fetish as a way of actively, and deliberately, creating new relations (2005: 407). He tells us that the artefacts we create with our human hands end up being the same things that we kneel down before and worship (2005: 411).

The problem with this statement is that through the idea of being 'social' we once again encounter the problem of anthropocentrism. Applied to religious statues such as the Virgin, I would develop this by suggesting that in the case of the Virgin of Alcala, this is better framed as a kind of 'creative tension' that exists between persons who are not social in the same way, but who become known and familiar in the presence of one another during encounters. Looking to Rosenthal's (1998) quote of Fo Idi, an Ewe Gorovodu priest, for support, the paradoxes that impose conflict on 'subject' and 'object' – that which is created and its creators – are only problematic when viewed from a particular, modernist angle. Fo Idi says, 'We Ewe are not like Christians, who are created by their gods. We Ewe create our gods, and we create only the gods we want to possess us, not any others' (Rosenthal 1998: 45). The power of these crafted gods is not in question. Once the problem of materiality is suspended, tensions can form significant and lively parts of religious devotional encounters that take place at Alcala where power is negotiated, rearranged and relationally born anew.

The actual crafting/fastening of religious artefacts is also important when exploring the dynamics of 'touch' and forms a significant part of the discourses that involve both animism and the fetish. From the devotional currency (offerings) found in the shrine, to the statue herself, crafting and active human creativity are both unique to this vernacular tradition, and supportive of more general Andalusian Catholic protocols. For example, it is estimated by a local historian in Alcala that the statue-body of the Virgin of Alcala was handcrafted by an unknown craftsperson from a cedar of Lebanon over 600 years ago. Inspired by Biblical references (examples: Psalm 92:12, 104:16, Hosea 14:5–6), many Christian statues are made from cedar. The physical form of the Virgin started as wood that was then shaped by human hands into a human effigy. This is not, however, 'art for art's sake'. Making a distinction between religious 'idols' and art, Gell tells us that 'Idols ... are not depictions, not portraits, but (artefactual) bodies' (1998: 98). 'Artefactual bodies' such as the Virgin are anthropomorphised. Do her features influence the ways in which she is touched by devotees? The potentiality of her personhood was, however, already present in the raw material of the wood which would have had its own history and biography. Ingold indicates that the physical properties of materials must be considered in order to have the 'full story':

> Thus the properties of materials, regarded as constituents of an environment, cannot be identified as fixed, essential attributes of things, but are rather processual and relational. They are neither objectively determined nor subjectively imagined but practically experienced. In that sense, every property is a condensed story. To describe the properties of materials is to tell the stories of what happens to them as they flow, mix and mutate. (2011: 30)

Or do they co-mingle? Acknowledging the raw materials from which the statue-body of the Virgin of Alcala was crafted not only adds another dimension to the story of her personhood, but begs further questions with regard to her material composition that cannot be easily answered. One might, for example, question how materials such as wood or stone are chosen to host religious identities. Is there some inherently recognisable quality in the wood chosen to become the Virgin of Alcala that her creator noticed? One might also inquire about the stages through which raw materials pass before they are capable of housing a deity, especially one that is perceived as inherently powerful. The answers to these questions can only receive speculation because the processes under which the Virgin of Alcala was crafted are unknown. Still, as the artefactual body of the Virgin exists, it is fruitful to consider the 'materials of her materiality' in that it adds an extra dimension to this chapter's discussion about 'touch' and crafting, the crafting of relations and the crafting of 'persons'.

Caretaking

Modalities of statue caretaking epitomise the dynamics of 'touch' in its most intimate form. After all, caretaking is also a form of crafting the invisible lines that constitute relations. There are two forms of vernacular caretaking at the shrine of the Virgin of Alcala. First, there is the care given to her by her principal live-in caretaker called the *Santero*. The *Santero* is a man who cares for the Virgin on a day-to-day basis. He is responsible for the upkeep of the shrine, and for her security. Second, within the cult of the Virgin, there is an elite group of roughly eight women called *camaristas*. These women, with their significant roles within the community, are responsible for ritually bathing and changing the clothes of the Virgin in accordance with the Catholic liturgical year. Since the Virgin is not only a gendered 'female' artefactual body, but a virginal one, accounts given by the *camaristas* revealed that it is strictly taboo not only for a man to see her disrobed, but for anyone outside of the *camaristas* (male or female) to be present during the changing.

These rituals, as well as the *camaristas* themselves, are said to carry an air of mystique in the village. Only women of a particular standing in the community are permitted to be *camaristas* and to touch the Virgin in what are referred to by them as 'beautiful, feminine, intimate moments'. Touching the Virgin in these moments of encounter takes on an intimate quality that is not commonly experienced by other devotees. These modes of 'touch' combined with the ways in which the statue is addressed, signal the animist potentialities addressed before, providing practical evidences about the ways in which personhood emerges through physical interactions. As will be discussed in the next section, caretaking, dressing, bathing, speaking with, crafting and giving gifts to a religious artefact such as the Virgin all fall within the performance category of 'to fetish'.

THE FETISH, 'TO FETISH': OFFERINGS AND DISPLAY

When material cultures are acknowledged as forming significant parts of religious contexts and experiences, discourses surrounding the fetish as both critical term and material object are never far behind. This is probably due to the fact that 'matter' has been very much distanced from academic pursuits for so long, that the fetish within animism is one of the only existing discourses that can be drawn upon with regard to combined issues concerning 'power and matter'. I will therefore begin this discussion of the fetish by acknowledging that the epistemological and cosmological differences between fetishists and vernacular Catholics are significant, and further, with the assertion that vernacular Catholics are not 'fetishists'. It is not my intention to turn the tables on Catholics and accuse them of doing and being that which early Portuguese tradesmen accused the African 'others' they encountered of doing, e.g. attributing power to inanimate, seemingly valueless objects while being unaware that the Portuguese's own amulets and crucifixes might have made their accusations appear suspect (Latour 2015: 91). As Pietz has pointed out, the critical use of the fetish, similar to animism, persists in causing theoretical and other problems for academics due to its 'sinister pedigree':

> Discursively promiscuous and theoretically suggestive, it has always been a word with a past, forever becoming 'an embarrassment' to disciplines in the human sciences that seek to contain and control its sense. (1985: 5)

It is, however, for this reason that the fetish warrants attention and discussion. Positively, Meyer tells us that the fetish is the epitome of material religion (2006, 2012). Other scholars, too, have picked up the fetish, dusted it off and found it useful in gaining better understanding of the roles of matter (e.g. Pels 1998, 2008; Graeber 2005; Manning and Menely 2008; Whitehead 2013a, 2013b). But what, exactly, is a fetish 'thing'? A few words must now be dedicated to unpacking this problematic so that we may better know the devil with whom we are dealing.

The material fetish is a thing born of relationships: relationships to place, relationships between persons, and relationships to whatever is present in the moment of its creation. From whichever angle we approach it, the fetish is born of 'touch'. It often conjures up unsettling images of hair, bone, stone, wood, plastics, mud and fingernail clippings. Although standard acceptance of the etymology of the word 'fetish' as 'that which is made' (Johnson 2000: 229) persists, there are other meanings, too. According to Latour, Charles de Brosses (who coined the word 'fetishism') 'in 1760, linked its origins with *fatum*, or destiny, the source of the French noun *fée*, "fairy", and of the adjective form in the noun phrase *objet-fée*, "fairy-object" (also of the English adjective "fey")' (Latour 2015: 89). Building on this, the word 'fey' in English signifies that which is feral, wild and savage – much like the material fetish object. As I have suggested elsewhere (Whitehead 2013a, 2013b), the fetish is an artefact which has the power to traverse worlds and boundaries, to heal, to protect, to make magic, to punish and to bind agreements. It also has the ability to mediate, transform and seal contracts. Similar to Catholic, Hindu or Buddhist statues found in static or portable shrines and temples, fetishes are dressed, fed and housed. The fetish is sometimes treated as a god; yet like the Virgin, it also stands at the mercy of its creators. Inanimate in appearance, the fetish is by no means static. It is functional and productive. Similar to Catholic rosary beads or amulets, the function of the fetish can be talismanic in that it offers protection; and similar to both the statue of the Virgin and to the offerings found at her shrine (especially those of hair or *ex-voto* limbs), the fetish is an extension of the fetishist.

The term fetish also has practical theoretical applicability. Johnson posits that we reinstate the fetish as a 'fluid, mediating term, an idea about objects, not an object itself – a mode of action, "to fetish"' (2000: 260). He says

> Fetish may be best viewed as a mode of action rather than a kind of object itself. It is a condensation of social powers onto an object in order

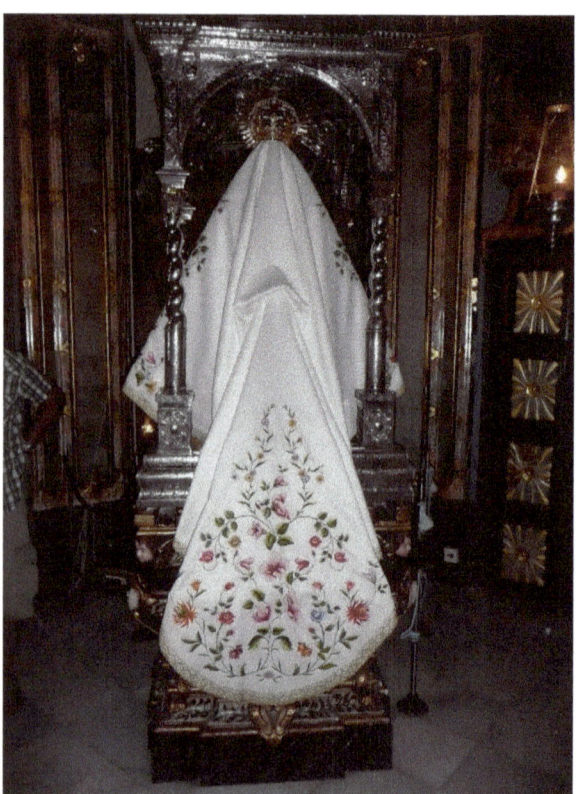

Figure 10.3 Under the white mantle. Photograph by Amy Whitehead.

to reconfigure them. 'To fetish' would therefore be more apt than 'fetish.' Viewed in this broad sense, it is a structuring technique of human consciousness in time, not an evolutionary stage of the false attribution of power to objects, a stage now surpassed. (2000: 249)

This advance whereby the fetish is considered in verb-form, e.g. 'to fetish', is here built upon and equated with 'touch'. Applied to the materialities and performances surrounding the Virgin, it can be argued that devotees 'fetish' in certain circumstances. This can be when they make, or give offerings, or when they go beneath the back of the Virgin's mantle and make a request (Figure 10.3). Although Johnson suggests that 'to fetish' is more apt than 'fetish', I am arguing that the fetish, in its flexibility, can be either object or verb, or both. Appropriate usage will depend on the nature of the performance in question. As previously established, the fetish is relationally viable, hardly static, and has a course of its own. According to Pels, the matter of the fetish 'strikes back' (1998: 91).

Offerings, sentimental value, display

'Touch' takes on another dimension when its dynamics are discussed in relation to religious offerings, especially sentimental ones. Typically, offerings that I have observed in the shrine comprise such things as gold rings, framed and braided locks of hair, and hospital bandages. They can also be photos of loved ones, medals, baby shoes, baby dummies, baby pictures and photos of babies in the shrine, bracelets, earrings, *ex-voto* paintings and drawings, cigarettes or pieces of cloth. In some instances the value of these objects is economic, normative of Western value structures, and obvious. Gold and silver jewellery are commonly seen in the shrine, for example. Yet the value of other offerings is personal, or *sentimental*, and remains a secret kept between devotee and Virgin. As with the measurability of the authenticity of rituals, or the processes by which religious statues are crafted, the intentions with which each of these offerings is given cannot be known. What is clear, however, is the fact that offerings of all description are visibly abundant in the shrine.

As demonstrated before, the diversity in function, usage and materials makes the fetish usefully applicable to examining the dynamics of 'touch', as in the case of the Virgin. In its flexibility it highlights the creative uses of a variety of materials in devotion and provides a theoretical premise from which to understand their complex roles. This assertion is best illustrated when working from the previously-mentioned etymology of the word, which is, 'that which is made' (Johnson 2000: 229). The fetish, like offerings, is a thing of creative relational engagement. As it mediates between 'persons' crafting new social relations within the 'relational zone' (akin to Graeber's 'fetish zone' [2005: 432]), its value and function shift and change according to needs, desires and intentions. This idea is best exemplified through looking at the roles of sentimental objects as extensions of devotees. Johnson says:

> In sum, if one means of reclaiming the fetish is tracing its etymology and usage, the other is by changing its arrow of valuation from denoting that which is Other to that which is right under our noses. That is to say, there may be social/cultural phenomena that are most usefully understood under the rubric of the fetish – phenomena whose primary criterion is their materiality and condensed signification. Obvious examples named above include a wedding ring or a photo of the beloved. (2000: 252)

This 'condensed signification' is relational and found in the sentimental objects given as offerings to the Virgin. Renfrew says, 'Often the term "sentimental value" is used to refer to the estimation that a specific person accords an object when the high estimation is not widely shared' (1986: 158). Renfrew's statement suggests that the value of sentimental objects is unique and cannot be replicated. Parallel to the fetish whereby their compositions are dependent on the materials available in the moment of their creation, this can be likened to the uniqueness of a fingerprint. No one devotee will have the same fingerprint, any more than one offering of sentimental value found in the shrine will have the same value as another. Moreover, it can be argued that sentimental objects of devotion are generative of a particular type of personhood where they are motivated to perform and be performed. In indicating that performances between human persons and object persons are co-created, Pels has noted that

> People perform objects ... but these objects also perform people by constraining their movements and by suggesting particular encounters between them and others. Similarly, in various ways, amulets, mascots and charms influenced the ways in which people behaved in certain situations, directly affecting how they experienced and navigated the world. (2003: 13)

So whereas protocols might be in place that indicate what the Virgin 'likes' to receive in terms of offerings, sometimes objects (especially sentimental ones) might have their own, unique agenda.

Discussions of 'things' that have sentimental value often involve the notion of 'essences', and 'essences' find their way into objects through being in a prolonged state of touch with their wearers. Echoing Frazer's idea of 'contagious magic' where 'things which have once been in contact with each other are always in contact' (1963 [1922]), the offerings that can best exemplify this idea are ones that have either (a) been a part of the family for years such as an heirloom or piece of jewellery, (b) bloodied hospital bandages, whereby bodily fluids will contain the essence of the giver, and (c) human hair. Other offerings, too, can be associated with this idea, such as photos; and this can be extended to the *ex-voto* images/plaster-cast limbs that line the walls of the shrine. The idea is that once an object has been in contact with a person or thing, it will have the ability to maintain a link or bond with that person or thing even when separated, and this makes these types of objects particularly potent when they become offerings. Pels says,

> Just as it would be imperialist to assume that magic is universal and fail to analyse its provincial meanings, it would be irresponsible to ignore that Frazer's homeopathic and contagious relationships can still help us understand why certain objects and images seem more powerful than others .... (2015: 122)

In the case of offerings of sentimental value given to the Virgin, once an object that has been in the possession of a devotee is given as an offering to the statue, part of the devotee remains in contact with that object and is therefore in constant and continual 'touch' with the Virgin. This can be seen particularly in the cases of jewellery (rings in particular) and locks of hair. Of course a hair offering can be considered a different type of object in that it is grown from a human body and is therefore a literal extension of a devotee. Yet when used as ritual or religious currency, it exemplifies another form of the 'co-mingling' discussed by Serres (2008), but with a difference. Once situated in the shrine, a part of a devotee's body will be in a state of continual touch with the Virgin and her protective, powerful context. These forms of expression, whereby 'things' once belonging to devotees such as rings of gold that are melted down to form part of the Virgin's crown are now 'forever' in physical contact or 'touch' with the Virgin, are responsible for maintaining ties with the Virgin. This exemplifies another way in which 'touch' works in religious contexts. Family and individual ties are created through the act of 'fetishing' and giving offerings to the Virgin whereby relationships with her are generated, renewed and maintained.

Display and the mantle

According to Hall, display and arrangement work 'like a language' (2003: 8). Designed to encourage 'touch', the Virgin's chamber is accessed via a winding staircase off to the side of the main altar display. Elevated at the head of the shrine, the Virgin of Alcala holds watchful sway over her 'court'. Pristinely dressed in her mantles darned in gold, she is displayed in such a way as to command a regal presence. Yet the Virgin is also displayed in such a way as to facilitate 'touch'. Deliberately accessible, 'the language' of display in the shrine of the Virgin of Alcala invites devotees 'to fetish'. Apart from the accounts given to me by the *camaristas*, I imagined that going under the back of the Virgin's mantle was probably the most intimate experience that a visiting devotee could physically have with the Virgin. Turner writes, quoting a female devotee of Mary who features a statue of the Virgin on her private altar:

> Most of us look at a statue or a picture and we know it's just that, but we don't want it to be just that. It's our link. Even though it's made out of stone, it's not just stone – it's spirit .... With Mary, I hope that she will someday envelop me physically, and take me in her robes. (Turner 1999: 115)

This desire to be taken into the Virgin's 'robes' (here discussed as 'mantle') is common for Marian devotees. For this reason, a statue whose display facilitates frequent touch may be more relationally capable of personhood than one who is cordoned off. If, as Hall (2003) suggests, display and arrangement 'work like a language', then it can be asserted that they have the ability to send out direct invitations to touch in some religious settings, while signalling where not to touch in others. Significant for this case study is the fact that 'going under the mantle' is the thing to do in relation to the Virgin. And this, I would assert, is responsible in part for the popularity that the Virgin of Alcala enjoys.

The presence of the rich material cultures and ensuing ritual performances that exist in and around the context of the shrine lend themselves to the creation of further relational possibilities. In an interview with the village priest, I was told that the Virgin's mantle is ritually blessed through a special mass before it can be placed on the statue-body. In line with this chapter's theoretical premise that offerings are extensions of devotees, it can be suggested that once blessed and placed on the Virgin, the mantle becomes an extension of the Virgin. Since this exploration into 'touch' considers the Virgin of Alcala, the 'mantle' can be likened to a first-class relic, e.g. a thing of the utmost importance to a saint. A second-class relic will be a part of a thing, such as a piece of cloth from a shirt. Third- and fourth-class relics are things that have been in 'touch' with first- and second-class relics. The class system within which relics find themselves is further demonstrative of the power of touch, contagious magic, and the ways in which matter can be theorised/understood using the fetish. Since the statue of the Virgin is small and stands on a pedestal, it is not easy for 'everyday' devotees to touch her statue-body. Further, her 'body' (apart from face, hands and feet) is mostly covered. The mantle therefore serves a valuable function to the Virgin's devotees and how they fetish. It is the point where tangible involvement 'happens', bodies co-mingle and, in the darkness, 'worlds' merge and new ones *emerge*. This type of physical, material involvement is made possible through the modalities of Virgin of Alcala's display, without which, I dare to venture, devotional practices would certainly decline and thus threaten the Virgin's very personhood, or her 'being'.

CONCLUSION

Critical usages of both the fetish and animism have framed discussions about the dynamics of 'touch' in this small-scale, yet richly colourful ethnographic detail of the case study of the Virgin of Alcala. The Virgin sits at the heart of community religious life in Alcala, and as demonstrated, she is engaged in a variety of performances that involve touch. Touch, it has been argued, is not only the medium through which this religion, and its religious performances, take place; it is the medium through which the animist personhood of the Virgin emerges, and the fetish – as both 'verb-like' action ('to fetish') and material object – is made viable and offered as a platform for critical explorations and discovery. Personhood is, after all, facilitated by touch during which times categories of subject and object mix, merge and 'co-mingle', giving way to the emergence of multiple ontological possibilities.

Establishing that the Virgin has a 'statue-body', caretaking rituals carried out by the *camaristas* have been explored, accounts of which signalled the more intimate dynamics of touch. The Virgin's feminine personhood informs, inspires and dictates the ritual performances in which she is touched. Crafting and creativity have also been considered, whereby the creation of artefacts and the materials used are explored as a means through which to understand further nuances of touch. The 'materials of the materiality' (Ingold 2011) have played a significant role in not only understanding the way in which the statue of the Virgin was crafted and made; but also in laying a foundation for explorations into both the material fetish and offerings. Offerings of sentimental value are found here to be of particular significance to this discussion about touch and the Virgin. Here, it is argued, touch is prolonged through objects being placed either on the statue-body of the Virgin, or within her shrine, that have been in long-term contact with a devotee. Touch, where 'essences' are involved and offerings are understood as extensions of devotees, is sustainable. This idea expands on animist understanding of personhood only being able to emerge in moments of active relational engagement where touch is fleeting.

These ideas are not only applicable to the study of the Virgin of Alcala, her materials/materiality, the offerings she receives and the devotional practices that take place in relation to her. Animism and the fetish, when used critically, are useful tools for scholars interested in exploring the dynamics, indeed the interfaces, of religion and the senses, particularly those that involve 'touch'. The material culture turn, along with studies in material, vernacular and/or lived religions, has signalled a move from focuses on that which cannot be seen, to the complexities involved in relationships and relational discourses: relationships that humans have with the world, with material cultures, with each other, and to/with statue-persons as in the case of the Virgin of Alcala de los Gazules.

REFERENCES

Barad, K. 2007. *Meeting the Universe Halfway: Quantum Physics and the Entanglement of Matter and Meaning*. Durham and London: Duke University Press. https://doi.org/10.1215/9780822388128

Boissevain, J. (ed.) 1992. *Revitalizing European Rituals*. London: Routledge.

de Witte, M. 2015. 'Touch' in Plate (2015: 261–266).

Frazer, J. 1963 [1922]. *The Golden Bough: A Study in Magic and Religion* (abridged edn). New York: Macmillan.

Gade, A. M. 2015. 'Emotion' in Plate (2015: 79–86).

Gell, A. 1998. *Art and Agency: An Anthropological Theory*. Oxford: Clarendon Press.

Graeber, D. 2005. 'Fetishism as Social Creativity: or, Fetishes are Gods in the Process of Construction', *Anthropological Theory* 5.4: 407–438.
https://doi.org/10.1177/1463499605059230
Hall, S. (ed.) 2003. *Representation: Cultural Representations and Signifying Practices*. London: Sage.
Hallowell, A. I. 1960. 'Ojibwa Ontology, Behavior, and World View' in S. Diamond (ed.), *Culture in History: Essay in Honor of Paul Radin*. New York: Columbia University Press. pp. 19–52.
Harvey, G. 2005a. *Animism: Respecting the Living World*. London: Hurst.
Harvey, G. (ed.) 2005b. *Ritual and Religious Belief: A Reader*. London: Equinox.
Ingold, T. 2011. *Being Alive: Essays on Movement, Knowledge and Description*. London and New York: Routledge.
Johnson, P. C. 2000. 'The Fetish and McGwire's Balls', *Journal of the American Academy of Religion* 68.2: 243–264. https://doi.org/10.1093/jaarel/68.2.243
King, R. 2005. 'Orientalism and the Study of Religion' in J. R. Hinnells (ed.), *The Routledge Companion to the Study of Religion*. Abingdon: Routledge. pp. 275–290.
Latour, B. 2015. 'Fetish-Factish' in Plate (2015: 87–94).
Leach, J. 2007. 'Differentiation and Encompassment: A Critique of Alfred Gell's Theory of the Abduction of Creativity' in A. Henare, M. Holbraad and S. Wastell (eds), *Thinking through Things: Theorising Artefacts Ethnographically*. London: Routledge. pp. 167–88.
Manning, P., and Menely, A. 2008. 'Material Objects in Cosmological Worlds: An Introduction', *Ethnos* 73.3: 285–302. https://doi.org/10.1080/00141840802323997
Meyer, B. 2006. 'Religious Sensations: Why Media, Aesthetics and Power Matter in the Study of Contemporary Religion', Inaugural Lecture, VU University, Amsterdam. 6 October 2006.
Meyer, B. 2012. 'Mediation and the Genesis of Presence: Towards a Material Approach to Religion', speech, Universiteit Utrecht, 19 October 2012.
Pels, P. 1998. 'The Spirit of Matter: On Fetish, Rarity, Fact, and Fancy' in P. Spyer (ed.), *Border Fetishisms: Material Objects in Unstable Spaces*. New York and London: Routledge. pp. 91–121.
Pels, P. 2003. 'Introduction' in B. Meyer and P. Pels (eds), *Magic and Modernity: Interfaces of Revelation and Concealment*. Stanford: Stanford University Press. pp. 1–38.
Pels, P. 2008. 'The Modern Fear of Matter: Reflections on the Protestantism of Victorian Science', *Material Religion: The Journal of Objects, Art and Belief* 4.3: 264–283.
https://doi.org/10.2752/175183408X376656
Pels, P. 2015. 'Magic' in Plate (2015: 117–122).
Pietz, W. 1985. 'The Problem of the Fetish, I', *RES: Anthropology and Aesthetics* 9 (Spring): 5–17. https://doi.org/10.1086/RESv9n1ms20166719
Plate, S. B. (ed.). 2015. *Key Terms in Material Religion*. London: Bloomsbury.
Renfrew, C. 1986. 'Varna and the Emergence of Wealth in Prehistoric Europe' in A. Appadurai (ed.), *The Social Life of Things: Commodities in Cultural Perspective*. Cambridge: Cambridge University Press. pp. 141–168.
https://doi.org/10.1017/CBO9780511819582.007
Rosenthal, R. 1998. *Possession, Ecstasy, and Law in Ewe Voodoo*. Charlottesville: University of Virginia Press.

Serres, M. 2008. *The Five Senses: A Philosophy of Mingled Bodies*. London: Continuum.
Smith, J. Z. 2005. 'To Take Place', in Harvey (2005b: 26–50).
Turner, K. 1999. *Beautiful Necessity: The Art and Meaning of Women's Altars*. New York: Thames and Hudson.
Tylor, E. 1871. *Primitive Culture* (2 vols). London: John Murray.
Whitehead, A. 2013a. *Religious Statues and Personhood: Testing the Role of Materiality*. London: Bloomsbury.
Whitehead, A. 2013b. 'The New Fetishism: Western Statue Devotion and a Matter of Power' in G. Harvey (ed.), *The Handbook of Contemporary Animism*. New York: Routledge. pp. 260–270.

Amy Whitehead is a MA tutor for the Sophia Centre for Cosmology in Culture at the University of Wales Trinity Saint David, UK, and Managing Series Editor for 'Bloomsbury Studies in Material Religion'. Her research focuses on the material and performance cultures of religion, including the dynamics of ritual and the relationships that ensue when power is understood as inherent in matter.

Index

aesthetics 37, 54, 138, 156
Africa and its diaspora 84-106, 181
ancestors 12, 37-60, 86, 89, 161, 181
animism 49, 54, 215-236
artefacts 125, 192, 215-236
auspiciousness 9-10, 52, 55, 57

belief, believing viii, 24, 49, 50, 56, 81, 84, 86, 104, 105, 112, 114, 117, 121, 131, 137, 138, 142, 143-144, 158, 196, 219, 221
Buddhists 37-60, 137, 228
Byzantium 13, 109-130, 212

Candomblé 13, 84-106
chanting 53, 120, 124
China 12-13, 37-60
Christians 4-5, 13, 14, 46, 56, 72, 102, 160, 163, 164, 165, 177-179, 181, 182, 185, 194, 215-236
clergy, priests 19, 20, 23, 27, 30, 31, 44, 45-46, 50, 56, 68, 71, 87-93, 120, 121, 154, 155, 157, 158, 161, 163, 164, 177, 192, 196, 203, 210, 216, 224, 232
confession 191, 200-208, 209, 210-212
cosmology 1, 3-9, 10, 28, 44-46, 75, 78, 80, 86, 87-89, 95, 96, 98, 99, 102, 104, 111, 114-120, 131-146, 222, 223, 227, 233

dance 6, 10, 41, 84, 86, 92, 103, 153, 155, 156, 164-165, 170, 172-175, 177, 181, 185, 208
darśan 131-146, 221

destiny 26, 87-89, 97, 126, 227
devotion 12-13, 38, 56, 84, 90, 91, 97, 112, 113, 118, 142, 143, 162, 181, 197, 210, 211, 212, 215-236
divination 10, 41, 87-89, 191
drone metal music 182-183
drums 11, 53, 89, 92, 170-188

Eleusinian Mysteries 13-14, 149-169
emotions 38, 39, 41, 54, 57, 135, 197, 221-222

festivals 9, 24, 39, 41, 43, 46, 51-54, 56, 63, 72-75, 77, 149-169, 170-188, 204
fetish(ism) 215-236
First Nations 13, 151, 170-188, 222
food viii, 5, 9-11, 13, 37-60, 63-83, 84-106, 133-134, 179, 201-202, 203, 219
funerals, wakes 53, 170, 177-179, 184, 216

gender vii, 10, 32-33, 73-75, 92, 96, 98, 103, 118, 131-132, 134, 138, 140, 146, 172, 174, 175, 176, 181, 186, 196, 200, 216, 218, 226, 232
gifts ix, 19-36, 37-60, 84-106, 135, 139, 141, 161, 184-185, 191-214, 217-218, 219, 224, 226
Gnostic Christians 164
Greece / Greeks 5, 13, 14, 23, 25, 30, 31, 109-130, 133, 139, 149-169, 191-214, 219

health and healing 9, 14, 23, 30, 39, 49–50, 54–57, 86, 97, 114, 144, 191–214, 216
Hindus 9–11, 77, 132, 140, 143–144, 228

icons 109–130, 180, 182–183, 185, 212
idolatry 112, 113, 114, 221
imagination 11, 65, 81, 113, 208
incense vii, 4, 7, 12, 12–13, 19, 30–32, 34, 37–60, 68, 120–121, 124, 133, 140, 216
Indigenous 13, 151, 170–188, 222
initiation 13, 88–91, 93, 143, 149–169
invisibility 6, 8, 13, 14, 46, 111–114, 117, 121, 127, 135, 156, 180–181, 195–196, 200, 208, 226, 233, 234
Israelites / Jews 4, 19–36, 123, 125

kinaesthesia 206

liturgy 85, 86, 94, 116, 118, 120, 124, 216, 226

Māori 7–8
Maya 6–7
meditation 2, 42, 50, 132–137, 141, 144
mediums 42, 44, 92, 93
Melanesia 180
Mesoamerica 6–7
Métis 13, 170–188
morality 10, 46, 48, 50, 141
Mount Gerizim 19–36
Muslims 10–11, 26–27, 140, 182
Mysteries 13–14, 75–80, 149–169

oratory, orator 3–9, 162, 165
Orthodox Christians 13, 109–130, 133

pain 3, 118, 123, 126, 159, 176, 181, 196, 203, 207–208
Paradise 5, 116, 118
piety 10–11, 12, 142
pilgrims, pilgrimage 12, 23–25, 44–46, 53, 158, 193–194
popcorn 97

possession ix, 92, 93, 181, 225
prayer 20–21, 24, 38, 41, 46, 47–48, 49, 54, 103, 118, 119, 175, 208, 210
preferences 63–83, 84–106, 112
processions 7, 12, 23–24, 98, 124, 153, 154–160, 164–165, 219, 224
prostration 7, 37–39, 54–56
protection 28, 49, 55, 96, 98, 118, 196, 216, 224, 227–228, 231
punishment / punitive 31, 118, 192, 201–208, 210, 212, 227
purity / purification 14, 49–50, 71, 102, 140, 154, 175, 181, 191, 194–196, 199–200, 211

regalia viii, ix, 11–12, 23, 33, 99, 126, 154, 170, 172, 175, 185, 226
restaurants 10, 51, 62, 104
rites of passage 86, 184, 196
Roman Catholic Christians 13, 86, 109, 113, 214, 215–236
Roman world 10, 13, 14, 43, 63–83, 112, 114, 191–214, 216

sacred / profane distinction 20, 24–25, 30, 31, 42–43, 45–46, 77, 84–85, 93, 121, 140, 162–163, 172, 180, 184–186, 193–196, 198, 204, 208
sacrifice 4–5, 19–36, 47–48, 64, 67–68, 73, 74, 76, 84, 85, 90, 92, 93, 126, 138, 153, 155, 158, 202, 203
Samaritans 19–36
sense of place ix, 8, 54
sex 32–33, 196, 203, 204
Sikhs 13, 131–146
silence vii, ix, 4, 6–7, 14, 93, 149–169, 178, 215
singing / songs vii, 3, 5–6, 33, 41, 86, 93, 120, 133, 134, 135, 138, 144, 149–169, 170–188, 224
Spanish 215–236
statues 11, 14, 45, 47, 52, 55, 57, 68, 123, 132, 137, 144, 154, 157–158, 191, 194, 197–198, 209, 211, 215–236
synaesthesia vii, ix, 67

taboo 30, 46, 77, 80, 87–89, 95, 99, 104, 112, 162, 191–193, 196, 203–204, 205, 212, 226
transformation 3, 42–43, 97, 118, 157, 181, 182, 197, 199–200, 212, 228
transgression 192, 201–205
Trobriand Islanders 180

trust 2, 9, 48–49, 210

value (sentimental) ix, 3, 51, 85, 99, 105, 114, 185, 227, 229–232, 234
violence ix, 4, 25, 66, 204

yoga 136, 141, 145

www.ingramcontent.com/pod-product-compliance
Lightning Source LLC
Chambersburg PA
CBHW061949240426
43669CB00052B/2969